OVERCOMING
DEAFNESS

The Story of Hearing and Language

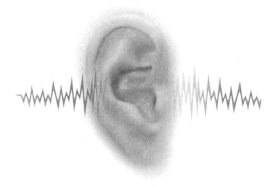

OVERCOMING
DEAFNESS

The Story of Hearing and Language

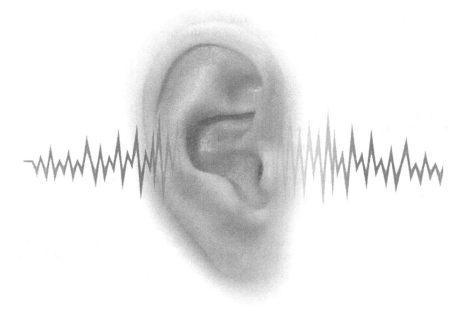

Ellis Douek

Guy's and St Thomas' Hospital, UK

Imperial College Press

Published by

Imperial College Press
57 Shelton Street
Covent Garden
London WC2H 9HE

Distributed by

World Scientific Publishing Co. Pte. Ltd.
5 Toh Tuck Link, Singapore 596224
USA office: 27 Warren Street, Suite 401-402, Hackensack, NJ 07601
UK office: 57 Shelton Street, Covent Garden, London WC2H 9HE

Library of Congress Control Number: **2014940263**

British Library Cataloguing-in-Publication Data
A catalogue record for this book is available from the British Library.

OVERCOMING DEAFNESS
The Story of Hearing and Language

ISBN 978-1-78326-464-3
ISBN 978-1-78326-465-0 (pbk)

Typeset by Stallion Press
Email: enquiries@stallionpress.com

Printed in Singapore

"Your tale, sir, would cure deafness!"

William Shakespeare
The Tempest

To Gill

Contents

Preface

Times Change

Louis de Bernieres' novel *Captain Corelli's Mandolin* begins with an old fisherman on a Greek island complaining of deafness in one ear. It is not clear what had brought him to the doctor after years of suffering. On inspection, the doctor saw a pea impacted in the fisherman's ear canal which must have been there since childhood as it was encrusted with wax and dirt. Since he had only a few tools, the doctor straightened a fishhook, poured water into the fisherman's ear to soften the pea, and literally fished it out.

The doctor took credit for curing the man but he did not mention the pea that was causing the fisherman's deafness as that would have provoked amusement and detracted from his success. The doctor's ingenuity and skill would have been unfairly brushed aside by hilarity if the details had been known. The doctor's reputation was enhanced and the islanders were comforted by his presence among them. The fisherman, who had never known anyone who had had an operation, enjoyed the attention. Nonetheless, the procedure could well have gone very wrong as damage can easily be caused to the ear when removing foreign bodies.

That incident took place before the Second World War, and though my own department at Guy's Hospital in London is now equipped with the most advanced technology, our feelings and anxieties are probably similar to those of the inhabitants of that tiny Mediterranean island, even if our expectations are not.

A Short History of Medicine and Disease

The concept of "infection" is relatively recent. Louis Pasteur, whose discoveries provided support for the theory of germs in diseases, could perhaps walk about the streets today without his dress attracting too much more attention than the odd double take. Yet even when he was an old man, many doctors and scientists still refused to believe in the existence of germs.

Western medicine is derived from Hippocrates and the ancient Greeks and codified by Galen, the Roman physician. Hippocratic medicine considered itself superior and enlightened because it did not accept the intervention of demons and magic. Disease was considered to be caused by an imbalance of the humours. This approach spread as far as India, presumably taken there by Alexander's invasions, where it still thrives today in its own form.

The medicine of ancient Babylon, on the other hand, was swept away contemptuously by the rationalists, both Greco-Roman and modern, because of its belief that disease was the result of infestations by demons. That dismissiveness may have been a disaster, and if today I were to discuss medical theory with an ancient Babylonian doctor, he would understand me well enough when I explained that we can now see these demons with our microscopes. I would tell him that they were not invisible after all, but were so small that they entered the body unseen, and that we called them germs. With a Greek doctor I expect I could only discuss the effects of stress on the balance of mind and body! Who knows how many epidemics might have been avoided, how many millions saved from death, if the Greeks had had some respect for these tiny demons and their capacity to hop from one person to another? Indeed the Babylonians suspected that they were contagious and advised families to get rid of the bedding of the sick as the demons may still have been lurking about. Interestingly, up until 1922, Public Health rules in the United Kingdom ordered that the bedding of those who had succumbed to consumption or tuberculosis be disposed of by burning

We now not only accept the presence of germs even though we cannot see them, but we give them names and can grow them on nutrient jellies. This has been particularly useful as we can place drops of different antibiotics on the jellies to see which of them kill the germs. It takes two or three days to discover what the germ is vulnerable to but at least we can use the right medicine. All these tests are done *in vitro*, which is Latin for "in the glass" and means that they are done outside the body on a specimen of infected tissue taken with a swab from the ear canal. This way we can choose to treat the patient either with antibiotic pills or with drops directly in the canal or both.

Aiding Hearing

When I was a medical student very little could be done to improve hearing. Hearing aids had only recently become available but electrical equipment had not yet been miniaturised and the source of power was the size of a car battery.

In the absence of antibiotics, childhood infections recurred every foggy and smoke-polluted winter, leaving many with perforated eardrums. As otosclerosis, a common inherited condition, was still inoperable, a large part of the population had diminished hearing. War trauma, epidemics and malnutrition had been the main concerns in the first half of the 20th century but then antibiotics and middle ear surgery together almost eradicated deafness resulting from the complications of chronic infection, glue ear and otosclerosis, which were by far the main causes of hearing loss. On the other hand, as life expectancy was around 66 years in men and slightly longer in women, deafness due to old age had yet to become a problem, and it is a measure of the success of modern medicine that deafness in old age is a problem only because our life span continues to extend.

When, by the year 2000, the cochlear implant allowed even those with total nerve deafness to hear a little, the last obstacle was pushed aside, so that virtually every type of deafness can now be cured by an operation or improved upon with an electric device.

Before these advancements in surgery and hearing aids, much had been done to understand the causes of deafness, long before any progress in surgery or the advent of hearing aids and that is what laid the ground to our present success. It is to the extraordinarily dedicated teachers who did so much to give the deaf a better chance that we are most indebted.

Communication

We know that animals communicate by chemical signals or pheromones, or by sounds, as evidenced in the multitude of animal calls. Bees carry out an elaborate dance along an axis which gives the direction of the nectar relative to the sun, while the rate at which they wiggle is a visual indication of the distance. Although all animals including humans can communicate without sound it has played the most important part in the development of language and of socialisation.

I suspect that the difference between communication and language is more than just one of degree but the definition of language continues to elude me. I suppose it is a system of meaningful words combined together grammatically in an infinite number of sentences allowing us to communicate what we wish. Language can be written or represented by gesture, but sound has always been the most important, most evidenced by the history of music and poetry. Music allows the composer to communicate feelings that words cannot express. Poetry, which uses both music and words, has a place in human communication so ancient that it predates literacy. It is important to remember that these forms of communication are as basic a means of human communication as a kiss or a caress.

Overcoming Deafness

Since the widespread use of the Internet we now have access to a wealth of information about hearing, from dedicated patient information websites and specialised articles to technical textbooks and manuals. The information can sometimes be intimidating rather than reassuring. This book is intended to provide an introduction to the history of hearing, the developments of the technology of hearing aids and common diseases of the ear. The subjects covered in this book are vast and there is much to interest those who cannot hear too well, who are concerned about ageing parents or who need to understand how a child develops speech. In other words, this book is for all of us.

Over my career as a doctor, we have managed to overcome deafness as there is now no one who cannot be helped at least a little. Since I have been personally acquainted with almost everyone involved, I can tell the story of overcoming deafness as my own.

The rapid technological advances that led to improved hearing was at odds with a vibrant signing but soundless culture and led, at times, to hostility. I could best come to terms with that by looking back as well as forward to a brighter future. I could understand the present only by including what happened in the past as that too is part of the story.

This book is concerned with sound, hearing and deafness as well as how we communicate by using sound and what happens when we are unable to do so. The ability to transmit our thoughts and feelings may be what defines our humanity and as music and poetry are an integral part of this process they are included by necessity in this discussion on communication and the story of overcoming deafness.

Acknowledgement

For a surgeon, undertaking a work that covers not only hearing but language, music and poetry, is daunting and requires encouragement so I am particularly grateful to Professor Larry Hench who first urged me to do it as well as to Dr Lawrence Buckman, Michael Stearns, Michael Gleeson and Professor Abraham Shulman of New York who all gave me support and confidence.

I also needed help, of course, which I received from the late Howard Milner and Joel Douek, both of whom illuminated music for me, while Beth Morchower Douek cleared up much about speech pathology and therapy. Nonetheless, only I am responsible for the conclusions I drew.

Alice Oven at Imperial College Press was an able supervisor and I quickly felt I could depend on Tasha D'Cruz, my editor, to protect me from errors. Gill, my wife, companion and friend listened continuously, read and advised.

Part I
Sound and Hearing

The sense of hearing allows us to perceive sound, contributing to our awareness of the environment, and to make use of it as a means of communication. We will describe what sound actually is and then what hearing is, the mechanism we have which makes us aware of sound.

Ancient records suggest that people have always thought a good deal about the nature of perception. Despite a lack of experimentation, it was generally understood that perception was associated with the identification of information about the environment. These physiological tools were categorized as five senses: sight, hearing, taste, smell and touch, and Aristotle discussed this process and its interpretation in *De Anima (Book II)*.

There are other types of data both internal and external, such as balance and proprioception, that are anatomically bound up with the sense of hearing and I have described them here. However, the way that the brain handles them is still problematic and Buddhists have long considered there to be another sense, that of the "mind", *ayatana*, manifested in the act of "mindfulness".

Western culture has kept the possibility of a sixth sense open and experiments bordering on science fiction have shown that implanted devices can allow the brain to "see" infra-red light. This means that there is no reason why any form of physical energy, including magnetc fields and radio waves, cannot one day be perceived though a brain implant. In theory, at least, we should ba able to hear high frequencies and even ultra-sound in the same way.

For the moment we are limited to the sense of hearing which invloves sensory cells that respond to vibrations of a particular range and their neural connections.

Chapter 1

Sound

Sound is the result of the oscillation of particles such as air. The frequency at which they vibrate decides if the outcome is sound. We have to know how to measure sound to understand it. Its two familiar aspects, loudness and pitch, can be measured relatively easily.

When I was a child we lived on an island in the middle of the River Nile where it flowed through the city of Cairo, separating the more urban side from its still somewhat agricultural districts which soon turned brusquely into desert. The island was considered particularly salubrious as the light breeze that followed the river was broken by our little land mass, creating a turbulence which, though slight by most standards, cooled the air in the heat of the day.

Our island was criss-crossed by wide, leafy streets and when we walked to school some tracts were still in cultivation. We wandered along irrigation channels and, faced with flat, tranquil water we felt a desire to shatter its stillness by throwing in pebbles to watch the ripples which formed around the point of impact.

We watched the little stones strike the placid surface giving rise to a circular wave that travelled outwards in all directions, forming what looked like a series of concentric rings.

The wave did indeed "travel" but in reality it was actually a movement back and forth of water particles creating alternating areas where they are compressed together followed by others of rarefaction as each particle nudges its neighbour then moves back. The wave that results from the movement travels away from the source, forming ripples, and gradually fades away as it loses its initial energy, getting weaker and weaker until it is hardly perceptible.

Apart from their strength or weakness, all waves have another characteristic, their length, which depends on the rapidity of the vibrations. A rather narrow band of wave-lengths, which lies between 20 and 20,000 to and fro movements or vibratory cycles per second, is rather special as we can hear them. Indeed, when particles of air vibrating within that particular range impinge on the eardrum, a thin taut membrane, it will follow their motion back and forth and give rise to the sensation of hearing. It is the vibrations that fall within those limits and which we can hear that we call *sound*.

The ear is not able to respond to vibrations that are much faster than 20,000, such as some we use in medical scans, so we cannot hear them and we call them *ultrasound*.

Vibrations that are slower than that range cannot be heard either, as they also have no effect on the ear but we can sometimes feel them and people have complained that low frequency vibrations from machinery have made them nauseous or ill. These slow vibrations are called *infrasound*.

Not everybody can perceive the whole range of sound frequencies equally well and as we grow older we lose the capacity to hear the faster vibrations. People over 60 years old rarely hear vibrations as fast as 10,000 vibrations per second and as we age further, our range becomes even more restricted at higher frequencies.

Sound vibrations may begin with a lot of strength or energy and we can hear them well as they set our eardrums in motion so we say they are *loud*. Eventually their energy reduces and the vibrations fade away until they become inaudible. An enormous amount of energy, like that produced by an explosion or even some disco loudspeakers, can be extremely loud and may even cause pain and damage the ear. This dangerous level of power is about ten times that of the minimum audible level.

As well as *loudness*, which depends on how strong they are, the vibrations have a different effect on our perception according to how rapidly the particles oscillate. Vibrations at a rate or frequency of 1,000 per second have a different effect from those at 250 per second. We hear a different sounds and say they have a different *pitch*.

If we strike a piano key it will make the string vibrate and in turn this will set in motion the particles of air around it and we will hear the sound when our eardrum vibrates with it. However, unlike the pebble in the water, the string continues to vibrate so long as it has enough energy so that the particles of air keep on oscillating at the same frequency as the string. The sound wave is not now a single event like the ripple in the water, which travels onwards but eventually fades away, but it is a continuous wave always maintaining the same rate of cycles per second.

The wave's frequency of oscillation remains the same and therefore its pitch does not alter. However, its loudness, which depends on energy that dissipates, gets weaker and the sound we hear becomes fainter. As the source of the sound, the vibrating string, repeats its disturbance of the particles of air at regular intervals with a definite frequency, the wave that results is called a *harmonic wave*, and the frequency is defined as the number of such disturbances or cycles per second. This regularity also means that the distance between similar points on the wave is repeated exactly and it is known as the wavelength.

Obviously the pitch, frequency and wavelength of the vibrations are closely related, and represent different aspects of the same thing.

One other aspect about sound waves to take into consideration is the fact that as the wave takes a certain amount of time to reach our ear, we have *speed of sound*.

Historically there was some understanding about vibrations but most thinkers thought that sound was merely a particle that went forward after being ejected from the source until it reached the ear. The Greeks knew quite a lot about vibrating strings and the Roman architect Vitruvius (1st century BC) made the comparison with the pebble in the water but it is not clear whether they understood how it was propagated. They certainly knew that sound travelled and that it travelled slower than light. They observed that a flash of lightning, a bolt from the heavens, perhaps thrown by a god, was seen instantaneously, whereas the sound it made took a little longer to be heard and that was the time it took the sound to travel the distance.

During the Enlightenment (a period so-called because people had begun to throw off the restrictions imposed on them by the Church and State) questioning nature rather than accepting it became more common. A French philosopher and mathematician called Galendi tried to imitate thunder using firearms. He measured the time between the flash and the sound of the explosion as well as the distance it had taken to reach him.

Considering the crudity of his methods, the conclusion he made regarding the speed of sound was surprisingly accurate. Due to technological advancements in this field, we now know that sound travels at around 332 metres (1,089 feet) per second.

Knowing the speed of sound was only a matter of scientific interest until the Second World War when experimental attempts showed that there was no reason why they should not fly at the speed of sound or even faster. Technology had begun to outstrip philosophical thought and scientific speculation as new materials and powerful jet engines became available. However, no one really knew what would happen should an aircraft fly at the speed of sound and there was only one way to find out. The first pilot to carry out the experiment was Captain "Chuck" Yeager of the US Air Force in 1947, aboard an aircraft he called *Glamorous Glennis*.

Those who took on the task of flying the plane at the speed of sound must have trusted the engineers who built the aircraft. When they actually reached the speed of sound (which was now called *Mach 1* after Ernst Mach who was born in what is now the Czech Republic when it was still part of the Austro-Hungarian Empire and worked on shock waves) the result was a dramatic bang. The loud bang was caused by the plane smashing through the particles of air which had become tightly compressed.

I remembering following these developments enthusiastically as a boy through inspiring films that told the story of those brave men. Today, their achievements are mostly forgotten although the potential ill effects of supersonic flight on the environment do generate interest and enthusiasm.

1.1 Measuring Loudness

"Loudness" is such a commonly used word that it seems unnecessary to question its meaning. Yet our descriptions of sensations depend on the language that we use.

We are fortunate with English: because it stems from so many different roots it has acquired an enormous number of words that are available to us.

I once attended a conference in Bordeaux where the organisers insisted I speak in French even though the audience was international, as the organisers had a good system of simultaneous translation. The French have their reasons about these things and I was anxious to cooperate.

During my presentation I could not find the French word for loudness. Colloquially they may say *"parlez plus haut"* or talk more "highly" which is unhelpful scientifically as the term "high" has to do with pitch rather than loudness. They could say *"fort"* which means "strong" but implies something different when speaking about sound. They might get around the problem by referring to volume but that, of course, has to do with space. In the end they have to say *"le 'loudness'"*!

English, on the other hand, is more flexible and we have permitted the word "loud" to wander into different meanings. For example, its basic meaning is "very audible" but it can also be used to mean an object that is garish or offensive as though it is shouting at you.

In measuring sound, it is important to note that we have different needs at different times.

Psychologists often use a system of ranking attributes using the values 1 to 5 and we can use this system to describe the loudness of a sound:

Just audible	1
Comfortable level for listening	2
Too loud for comfort	3
Unacceptably loud	4
Painful	5

This system is simple and is used in numbering the volume control of many hearing aids, usually with the advice that our patients to keep it on number 2.

Not everyone would be happy with this system. The manufacturers of equipment, for instance, require great precision and may be uneasy at having 1 as the threshold of audibility as people are not identical. Nonetheless their equipment has to be standard.

In the earliest days of the Industrial Revolution, James Watt invented a machine that worked with the power generated by steam. He sold it to his clients by suggesting that they could replace a dozen horses by its use and so the power of the machinery is referred to as 12 horsepower or 12 hp. When machines replaced men rather than horses they could have used "manpower", but they did not.

Now power comes from such diverse sources that it would be out of place to describe a light bulb, for instance, as having horsepower. So we have given new names to our units. Unsurprisingly we call them "watts" after James Watt himself.

The intensity needed to produce a barely audible sound is described as the force exerted by 0.0000000000001 watts over an area of 1 cm^2! It would be better to stick with 1.

The pain level (our loudness, 5) works out at 0.01 watts per square centimetre which is 10,000,000 times greater than 1.

We cannot use such scales in everyday language as most of us prefer to refer to sound as being twice as loud or ten times as loud. In doing so we are talking about a "logarithmic" scale. We may have forgotten what that means but it is exactly the scale needed in this context.

The watt was dismissed as a unit to describe sound because of its unwieldiness. The new logarithmic unit was named the "bel" in honour of Alexander Graham Bell, the Scotsman who invented the telephone and founded the Bell Telephone Company.

An increase of 1 bel means that the loudness is ten times greater and 2 bel would make it ten times ten or a hundred times. These numbers are still too big for most of our needs so we use one tenth of a bel as our basic unit. We call it a decibel and write it as dB.

The loudness of a sound is therefore, for practical purposes, measured in *decibels*.

1.2 Measuring Pitch

If a sound particle oscillates back and forth in one second we can say that it vibrates at a frequency of one cycle per second.

The pitch we know as middle C is produced by vibrations of 512 cycles per second. This is how pitch was referred to for a long time but, just as "watt" became the measure of power, named after its discoverer, we now measure pitch using "Hertz" (Hz), after the German physicist Heinrich Hertz. Middle C then, should be called 512 Hz, while a tone of

1,000 cycles per second is 1 kilohertz (kHz). Although it is worthwhile commemorating the great men of science in this way, I find it helpful to remember that when we talk about Hertz we mean that particles are vibrating at so many cycles per second and produce a wave accordingly.

Although we reckon that the sound spectrum lies between 20 Hz and 20 kHz, when we come to our everyday life we are concerned with the part of the spectrum that allows us to hear, thus making speech intelligible, and to enjoy listening to music. That is why when we record hearing loss we do so only over the frequencies from 125–8,000 Hz.

1.3 Mysteries

It seems obvious that if there are no particles to vibrate then there can be no sound and that empty space, therefore, can only be totally silent. I believe this is true in practice, and that astronauts cannot shout at each other across space, but I am told that, in theory, things are more complicated. Waves are not all they appear to be, as quantum theory suggests that transmission takes the form of discrete little packets of energy or of some other physical property. Energy may even exist as tiny strings and that the universe is not empty at all but full of *dark matter*.

Then there are also Black Holes, mysterious objects that suck in matter but do so in a pulsatile manner causing gigantic ripples in space and equating to sound waves of 30,000 light years.

According to the Institute of Astronomy at Cambridge there is a huge Black Hole about 250 million light years away, in the constellation Pegasus which has probably been humming B flat for billions of years. The deepest note ever detected in the universe is about 57 octaves below middle C, even though its intensity is comparable to human speech.

These findings may well change our understanding of waves, including sound waves but until further exploration is done, the current rules on sound waves still apply.

1.4 How Sound Behaves

The "image" that the sound around us produces is both complex and chaotic. When we walk down crowded streets and visit supermarkets we are bombarded by visual, olfactory and acoustic stimuli. If we are familiar with the environment we will recognise some of these stimuli, even if it is only at the subconscious, and we become immediately aware of new ones.

As we move around, the sounds shift and contribute to our awareness of where we are, but as hearing is only one of the senses that come into play automatically in this process, it is difficult for most of us to separate one from the other. We just "know" where we are and what is around us. It is only when one of these senses fails us that we recognise its importance.

The Indian writer Ved Mehta, who was blinded at the age of four, gives a very moving description of his childhood in his book *All For Love*.[1]

> … I made sounds visible; their images resonating with the visual impressions stored away in my early memory… There were other aural signals. The echo in a room announced the furniture it contained. I would walk along the street with my hand in my mother's, astonishing her by counting the street lamps … a sort of sixth sense that the blind develop to perceive objects and terrain through, as it were, sound shadows, rather like a bat's echo-location system.

This perception depends on sound bouncing off objects. The sound is affected by an object's size, by whether it is close or distant, and its relation to the terrain. Blind people unconsciously sort out, classify and interpret these echoes in order to orient themselves and negotiate their way. Although this auditory vision is more acute in the blind, it can be acquired by training and in fact we all have this vision to some extent.

A person with poor hearing will suffer considerably as a result, and in a crowded and noisy situation it would be worse, even without attempting to listen to a conversation. We should not underestimate the problems that people who have only one good ear experience. In theory, they should hear perfectly adequately. In practice, the difficulty in localising the source of sound means that they can find it a disturbing and intangible world. Children who suffer in this way find it very difficult to tell where a sound is coming from in the classroom, and where the teacher is standing, if they cannot see her.

---

[1]Ved Mehta, *All For Love* (Granta Books, London: 2001).

My younger brother was deaf in one ear and we often discussed his problems. He had learnt to control his environment to a great extent by rearranging the chairs at meetings and knowing where to position himself but he told me that when surrounded by a crowd he would feel uncertain.

The design of buildings is very important to the way sound behaves but the way people react also varies. I once went to a fashionable restaurant with a group of friends where we found that we could not hear ourselves speak. As I could see that the problem was a simple one caused by many mirrors and other reverberating surfaces, I wrote to the management offering my services to attenuate this free of charge. The reply was an amusing letter explaining that they had already consulted experts on how to make the place noisier as that gave a buzz and made the place trendy. They also sent a list of quieter restaurants which they recommended.

Designing concert halls is an art form since the way sound behaves in a particular building favours the performance of particular types of music. For instance slow monophonic Gregorian chants are best suited to the reverberating Gothic cathedrals whereas smaller churches with shorter reverberation time favours polyphonic music. Atonal or twelve tonal music, such as some pieces by Schoenberg, are at their best with the least reverberation as in a recording studio.

As an experiment, I decided to test out the experience of music in different sized music halls, after so many of my patients complained of not being able to hear well at the theatre, particularly when the halls.

I thought I would start at the beginning, in the amphitheatre at Epidaurus, near Athens, which dates from the 5th century BC. Theatre festivals are held there in the summer in the open air to wonderful acoustics (though it is wise to bring a cushion to sit on the uncomfortable stone benches). I was familiar with this type of amphitheatre and I had heard open-air opera at the Verona Arena, a Roman amphitheatre, parts of which date from 30 AD. Amphitheatres had originated with performances in ancient Greek times when the audience sat on hill slopes where the acoustics had, by chance, been found to be particularly good. Formal seating was later added and the setting for performances became more permanent. By the Roman times many such theatres were built all over the empire, with stone tiers reproducing the original hillsides.

At Epidaurus the guide made us climb up to the uppermost terraces and, when everyone was still, he dropped a small coin where he was standing right at the bottom. Even though I was irritated by his melodrama as I had seen it all done before, I could not but be struck yet again by the extraordinary clarity of the sound. Later some of the actors who were performing there told me that although the acoustics were exceptional during an actual performance it was difficult during rehearsals in the empty arena because of the reflection and reverberation from the stone surfaces. The human body is very absorbent of sound as energy and retains more than two-thirds of the energy; this is therefore the most important factor in any theatre.

There has been little change in the basic facts of acoustics since Greco-Roman times. Indeed, it must undermine contemporary architects anxious to make their mark on our world by trying out exciting new materials, only to be told that they can do no better than to reproduce structures 2,000 years old. For one thing, in Northern Europe at any rate, the inclement climate is such that open-air Roman arenas such as those found in Jerash, Arles or Carthage are no more useful than open-air cinemas.

One main problem facing architects is that covered halls rarely have enough space to build the tiers and terraces that were naturally present in the open air amphitheatres of Greece and Rome. However, tiered seating is not a necessary requirement for most musical performances. In fact, the ceiling of a covered hall has the added bonus of reflecting sound onto the audience sitting on a flat horizontal floor.

When the Barbican concert hall in London was being commissioned, I was part of a test audience. There was a surreal quality about this experience as they went through the motion of sending us real tickets, even though they were free, and having ushers at the doors as in normal performances. The London Symphony Orchestra was conducted by Claudio Abbado and soloists such as Rudolf Serkin played. In normal circumstances these would have been important and highly publicised concerts; instead as we entered the dark and as yet unopened building there was an air of mystery. A secret concert was taking place.

The hall itself had been attractively furnished with a good deal of polished wood, carpet and fabric-covered seats. It had a floor sloping forwards towards the stage giving it an amphitheatre-like structure and there was also an overhanging balcony. Our job as the test audience was to see the effect of a concert with the audience in place rather than in an empty hall.

We took our seats in anticipation but as soon as the music started we were appalled. The sound was unacceptable. We looked at each other in dismay. Here was the symphony hall we had waited decades for, which had cost so much and which now gave us such poor acoustics.

The organisers were not at all worried as they knew it was a matter of adjustment, of reflectors here and there or vents to trap sound. That was why we had been invited to come in the first place. At the interval we changed our seats and after a few such episodes we got quite good at commenting on the quality of the sound. What I found most interesting was that as everything got gradually better, people became more finicky and also showed different predilections. Some preferred it when the strings were given greater prominence, some liked a crystal-clear definition while others preferred a more blurred and blended effect.

I have often since wondered what it is that gives an overcrowded and expectant hall the advantage over a half empty one. Obviously the psychological effects on both audience and players must provide the major part but I suspect that the acoustics themselves also have a role in the nature of the emotions engendered.

We are not surprised that a play involving two actors could hardly be performed successfully in a vast Gothic cathedral. Nevertheless concert spaces need to be designed with some degree of flexibility, as they often have to provide for a relatively wide repertoire from symphonic music to solo players. They need to be able to accommodate great choirs as well as small ensembles if we are to make full use of our halls. I learnt from my experiences at the Barbican that it is difficult to account for personal taste and that some people will always prefer one hall to another. With time, people become attached to the acoustics of particular halls even though they may technically leave quite a lot to be desired; of course, emotional memories also come into play as preferences are developed.

The hall itself selectively enhances or absorbs frequencies so that instruments do not sound the same if played in a room by themselves. In that sense the hall can be seen as an extension of the orchestra and the conductor who knows its properties can almost play it as an instrument, increasing the volume in the bass, for instance, or encouraging the higher frequencies.

When looking for the best conditions for listening in any environment there are three major considerations: the background noise must be right, the sound we want to hear should be loud enough and it should be adequately distributed.

1.5 Background Noise

Background noise in itself is not a bad thing. A completely dead, non-reflecting, soundproofed room offers a very unpleasant experience. Although we may not be happy in a restaurant that is so noisy that we cannot hear our companions, one so silent that we are forced to listen to other tables' conversation or the hum of the air conditioning is not ideal either. In a restaurant the buzz of conversation is attractive and can ensure privacy.

It is taken as a given now that there should be an absence of noise in a concert hall, where we are reminded at the start to switch off mobile telephones and where a cough is felt to be out of place. However, this was not always the case. It is only since the middle of the 20th century that classical concerts have been formal, almost church-like, as they are now. Prior to that, audience members walked about during a performance, ate, drank, chatted and even played cards. There were ways around this: Richard Wagner forced his audiences to concentrate on the music by extinguishing the lights and the Milanese at the Scala had to wait for Arturo Toscanini, the conductor, to get their audiences under control. At the other extreme, Sir Thomas Beecham (of the pharmaceutical firm that produced Beecham's powders) virtually employed the orchestra himself and thus had great authority over the performers. His authoritarianism extended as far as the audience and he would browbeat anyone who so much as sneezed.

Of course there is much to be said for our present formality and strict silence at classical concerts, but if this reverence were imposed on pop concerts it would spoil the fun.

Only a few decades ago considerable importance was attached to a symptom described by some deaf people who claimed that they could hear better in background noise than in the quiet. The symptom was given the name "paracusis" but no one seemed to understand the phenomenon.

The most dramatic description of paracusis that I have found was a 17th century one of a husband who had hired a drummer to follow his wife around beating his instrument to produce a low-pitched rumble whenever she wanted to talk to someone.

I think that today few believe that there really is such a symptom and that the patients benefit from others having to raise their voices to overcome low frequency noise.

1.6 Loudness and Sound Distribution

It goes without saying that a shy person who looks down and mumbles does not help the listener and a speaker who cannot project his voice is a bad lecturer (although the microphone has been a great boon to alleviate the situation).

Electric amplification is so widely used that many would be surprised to know that what they take to be "natural" sound in a concert setting is really the result of amplification from microphones placed a few feet above the source. The Royal Festival Hall in London used this amplification technique for a while but many people were dissatisfied with the original sound which was too "dry".

As previously discussed, the way sound is distributed depends on many things such as the size and shape of the room, the people and structures within it, the presence of reflecting surfaces and the nature of being enclosed or in the open air. The feeling that a room is "cosy" owes a lot to its visual appearance and to the memories it recalls but attention should also be given to the way conversation, with its raised voices, its whispers, its laughter and asides, sounds in the room.

I knew a couple who once decided, while in their late middle age, to move to an apartment which they furnished in an aggressively minimalist style. They gave no explanation for this (although I am sure a number of psychological factors were involved) but it made all their friends uneasy and none of them liked it. They referred to it as "clinical" and "cold" and I found myself paying special attention to the way voices sounded in their new environment. This left me convinced that the acoustic effects had much to do with the sense of unease most people had described though not a single person had commented directly on the sound. Everyone had pointed out the flat white reflecting surfaces and the lack of furniture only in visual terms.

The baroque decorations, curlews and angles so typical of old theatres and halls were often important in distributing sound. When 20th century tastes turned to minimalist and "functional" features, the terms were expressed mainly in visual terms and the resulting acoustic effects were very bad. It took considerable efforts to add shapes which work from the sound point of view without offending the modern eye. Our modern architects are to be once again disheartened to accept that ideal structures are based on concepts which are thousands of years old and on the interior decorations of the 18th and 19th centuries.

From the audience's point of view, their position within a concert hall or theatre is of importance. A general good guide is to position oneself within sight of the performers: generally speaking, if you can see, you can also hear. Seats at the back under a long balcony give poor sound and impair the hearing. At best a balcony should slope towards the front and have an adequate opening to the stage.

All these problems and their solutions are related to reflection and reverberation. Sound coming directly from the source, whether voice or instrument, dissipates quickly so that by the time it reaches the ear its energy is less than a 100,000th of what was produced even if the listener sits in the best seats. By the time it reaches the back it may be as little as a 10,000,000th of the original.

On the other hand the reflection from one surface to another enhances the sound. The early reflection should take less than 30 milliseconds; if it is more than 70 milliseconds then it will be heard as an echo.

Early reflection, particularly from the sides rather than the ceiling, gives an "intimate" feel as what we perceive is that the walls are nearby, more like a room than a hall. Different frequencies tend to behave differently too as carpets absorb high frequencies and reflect low ones while the opposite is the case with glass. Concrete and stone tend to reflect everything.

When decorating a room we tend to consider the visual aspects exclusively and this sometimes results in dissatisfaction though we may not know the reason why. If we want reflecting surfaces such as mirrors but are made to feel uncomfortable by the outcome, considering the acoustics may help restore the atmosphere by adding carpets or placing objects and furniture appropriately.

Another feature of sound in enclosed spaces is reverberation. This builds up as sound waves ricochet from everywhere and then decay in intensity. Naturally it depends on the size of the room as the greater this is the longer the reverberation time. The sound absorption of the furnishings also makes a difference, varying with fabrics as well as with the number of people present.

A long reverberation time increases the blending of the sounds and is favourable for music. A short reverberation time tends to give a lifeless feel that lacks depth while a long one gives a sense of the "big sound". In the theatre short reverberation results in a dry feel and is said to produce more definition.

Different types of music will do better in different acoustic environments and it is said that the availability of these spaces encourages the composition of particular pieces. Debussy's *La Mer* for instance needs a long reverberation time and the composer could only conceive the idea if there is an appropriate space where he can imagine its performance.

As a final note on sound, space and performance halls, I am often asked which seats one ought to aim for during a concert and my advice is usually to sit about 60 feet from the stage and off centre.

Chapter 2

Hearing

We need to consider the structure and function of the hearing mechanism and how each part is tested. Small children pose problems with testing hearing but it is particularly important to know how well they can hear.

2.1 The Mechanism of Hearing

2.1.1 *Evolution and development*

Many abnormalities of the ear are the result of errors during its development. Understanding the process of the development of the ear was necessary before dealing with the cure.

Even very primitive creatures such as worms which crawl in the ground may respond to vibrations. Some may even be sensitive to the range that we call sound but I doubt that they "hear" in the sense that we do.

For a creature to perceive that particular and useful range of frequencies, specialised organs have had to evolve. Some insects may be sensitive to only a very narrow frequency range. A cricket, for instance, can only hear a high-pitched zizzing sound with a frequency of 6 kHz, which it produces by rubbing its legs together. It uses it as a call in the mating process and does not seem to need to hear anything else. A tiny fly that lives contentedly in symbiosis on the cricket also relies on being able to perceive the same frequency so that it can find the cricket, but it too does not need to hear anything else. Two creatures, then, have evolved who neither can nor need to hear more than one tone.

Nature tries to be economical and will not waste itself on organs that are not needed. As evolution takes place in response to the pressures of survival, it takes account of changes such as climate and availability of food. This means that structures and organs, which were very useful to creatures living in an aquatic environment, could be dispensed with as they move to the land. New structures too, may be required to take advantage of the change but it is more economical to salvage unwanted parts of the anatomy and modify them, putting them to a different use, than to create totally new ones out of nothing.

Considering "Nature" and "Evolution" in this way as though it were not only a thinking entity but also a responsible house-keeper, hardly corresponds with reality but it is a useful convention. Organs do change from one species to another as thousands of years go by and vestiges of old organs remain, even if it is not use. Additionally, a particular organ, rather than disappear if it ceases to be needed, may evolve to be used for a different purpose.

Animals start to develop as three layers of a tube (Figure 1). Pits form as indentations in the outer layer of cells, which among other things, will

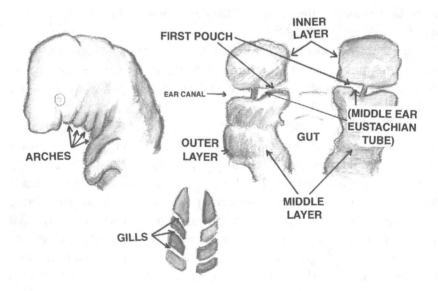

Figure 1.   A three-layered tube forms gills on the way to becoming an embryo.

become the skin, while pouches will bulge out of the inner tube, which will end up as the gut. For some embryos, such as the earthworm, that may be as far as it goes. A human embryo, on the other hand, will grow and change until it attains its final complexity, but the way it does this, twisting and folding, cells migrating in this direction or that follows a carefully preordained order.

Biologists have long realised that the path this pattern follows is itself like a journey along the memories of our ancestral species. Structures present in primitive fish appear only to be modified into those of archaic amphibians. These in turn may vanish completely or parts of them may grow to offer some unexpected if useful function in our own anatomy.

Primitive fish have a cartilage skeleton that includes plates around the mouth, which will evolve into the chewing apparatus of modern fish. Not all these structures are necessary in later species, but rather than disappear they alter in shape, become ossified and end up as the little bones that are part of the hearing mechanism in our own middle ears.

It is a moot point as to whether fish "hear" but they are certainly sensitive to vibration. This sensation comes from plaques at various places in the skin made of little bundles of cells which have a hair-like structure sticking out into the water (Figure 2). Mechanical vibration will bend these hairs and when they do, an electrical impulse is generated which travels along a nerve to inform the brain.

A fish has little in the way of landmarks to wend its path through water and it relies on such sensory structures to make it aware of the currents and movement of the water.

They have developed a specialised organ called the *lateral line*, which may be a canal or groove along the side of the body with the little clusters of hair cells along its way bending as the water flows by.

The fish also had to develop some way of keeping its equilibrium and this seems to have evolved from the front part of the lateral line which becomes embedded in the bone of the skull.

Our world is three-dimensional so if the fish is to have a sense of balance and location a single sensitive line along the side of its body is hardly sufficient. It would need three such canals, each in a different plane (Figure 3). This system could then respond to the flow of water in every

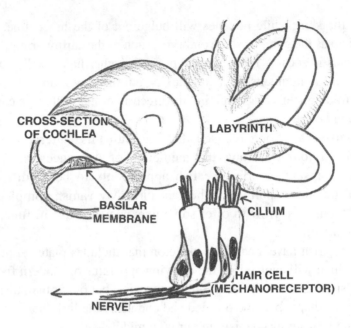

Figure 2. Mechanoreceptor (hair cell).

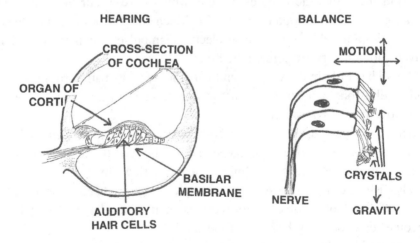

Figure 3. Sense organs in the ear.

direction so that the fish is aware of where it is going. Two further swellings form at the base of these canals which contain hairs, one in the horizontal and one in the vertical plane, so that the fish knows its position relative to the world and whether it is upside down or not, even if it is still.

The water enters the canals through one or more openings. However, when these creatures climbed from the sea onto dry land these openings closed, leaving this collection of semi-circular canals and swellings containing sensory hair cells isolated in the bone at the side of the skull. Some of the cells specialised in secreting fluid to fill the system, which is very similar to the original seawater.

For land animals, hearing was an advantage, and the organ of equilibrium and movement sensation became modified so that it could sense sound vibrations too. An extension of the sense organ appears in the form of a tube that ends blindly. The tube needs to be rather long in order to house the large number of hair cells that respond to the sound vibrations of a range of frequencies. To save space, the tube coils up like a seashell. We call the tube the *cochlea*.

The nerve fibres that lead from the hair cells serving both senses form into bundles and transmit their impulses to the brain, but as these are electrical they have to be insulated from each other, just as in any electric wire. This is performed by specialised cells called *Schwann cells*, which produce an insulating sheath as they grow along with the nerve fibres. It is from excessive activity of these cells that the tumour of the ear called the *acoustic neuroma* occasionally develops in later years. Furthermore, it is the failure of insulation that results in problems associated with multiple sclerosis.

In this way the animal kingdom evolved the inner ear to serve both *hearing* and *balance*, but there was more to come. This organ is embedded in the skull and can sense sound vibrations well if applied to the ground. However, it is a poor sensor for receiving sound vibrations from the air. Nevertheless, another change happened at the same time, by which nature was able to rectify this difficulty.

Fish, of course, breathe by filtering water through their gills. These gills were formed by slit-like indentations in the surface skin and out-pouches joining them from the inner tube of the primitive embryo. Water enters the pharynx by the mouth and is then forced out through the membrane between the pouch and slit. During this process oxygen is taken in and carbon dioxide bubbled out, resulting in the exchange of gases we call *breathing*. There are usually five gills separated by arches of cartilaginous tissue called *branchial arches*.

On land a different air breathing mechanism evolved using the lungs, making the gills redundant. By and large, the gills closed up and disappeared; but some elements were salvaged. It is possible to see the shape of the gills forming in the human embryo and then fading away, although not completely.

The opening of the first gill slit remains, and becomes the ear-hole. Around this opening a collection of little bumps form and by five months into the pregnancy they have become a human-looking ear.

The first pouch, which had grown towards the first gill, remains as a cavity in higher animals, becoming the middle ear and Eustachian tube, which opens at the back of the nose.

The bony tissue of the first branchial arch breaks up to form part of the chin, the cheek bones and the little bones of the sound-conducting mechanism of the middle ear, though some tissue from the second arch is also included there.

The ear canal is now separated from the middle ear cavity by only a thin membrane, which becomes the eardrum. These structures join the inner ear and its nerve, functioning well before the baby is born.

However, things, as usual, can go wrong.

A little boy presented with a severe developmental defect. He had no ears and no ear-holes. There were other unusual, though less dramatic features. He had a very small chin which in itself is hardly rare, and his eyes tended to slant downward at the sides as his cheek bones were also not well developed.

His abnormalities indicated a pattern suggesting a failure of the structures of the first arch to develop fully.

The boy's mother, who was Norwegian, brought me photographs of ancestral portraits going back a few generations. They were an important family many of whom were teachers, judges or preachers and had all risen to eminent positions. You could tell they were related as they all had the small chins and eyes which slanted downwards and outwards associated with the first arch.

This showed how such a developmental abnormality could be the result of inherited genes but also how it could be expressed to a degree varying from a distinctive family appearance to a severe defect that included deafness.

Some drugs can also interfere with the development of the embryo. Thalidomide wreaked havoc in the 1950s and ever since then we are very careful which medicines we allow pregnant women to take.

Rubella or German Measles, which is caused by a virus, can damage the foetus very badly, particularly in the early months of pregnancy. It affects the development of the hearing mechanism as well as other systems such as vision and the heart. Since vaccination has become widely available, these abnormalities have greatly diminished but it indicates that infections in pregnancy, perhaps with unknown viruses, can be responsible for developmental abnormalities.

Despite these possible slips, the development of the foetus generally works well enough and we end up with a structure of such intricacy, both in appearance and function, that the term beauty can be applied.

2.1.2 *Structure and function*

The *hearing mechanism* (Figure 4) consists of the ear, the nerve of hearing and its pathways and connections deep into the brain, which awakens our consciousness to sound. As we discovered in the previous section, the *balance mechanism* is also part of the ear.

Most people regard the *outer ear* as that which we can see sticking out of the side of the head and the *inner ear* as those parts which are out of sight.

In some ways this distinction between outside and inside is not unreasonable as an external problem appears to be mainly cosmetic while that of the inside involves the hearing mechanism itself.

From the point of view of disease and diagnosis as well as anatomy, however, the ear is best divided into three parts rather than two. The outer ear consists not only of the visible ear, or *pinna* to give it its Latin name, but also the ear-hole and canal down to the drum. It developed in the embryo from an invagination of the outer skin. Disease of this area may

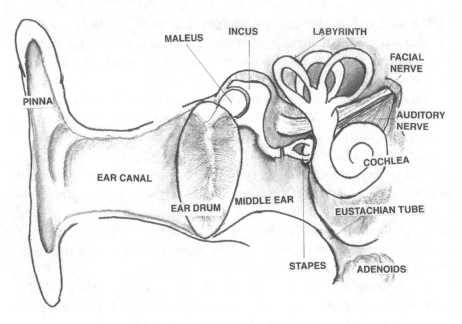

Figure 4. Structures of the ear.

be very unpleasant and painful but it is only very rarely serious and may not affect the hearing in the long run.

The middle ear, the air containing the cavity on the inside of the ear-drum, includes the tiniest bones in the body, called the *ossicles*. These bones connects with the back of the nose by the *Eustachian tube*. The middle ear and tube evolved from the first pouch formed from the embryonic pharynx. Disease in this area may be serious, even fatal, and will certainly affect the hearing, perhaps severely. Nevertheless, we are now usually able to treat this area very successfully.

Finally there is the real inner ear where disease is rarely life threatening but it is closely associated with the nerve and the brain.

2.1.2.1 *The outer ear (pinna)*

The pinna is made of elastic cartilage covered in skin. It is there because it has a role in collecting sound and directing it towards the ear-hole, particularly when it is a quiet sound. It is easy to test this by simply cupping the hand around the ear, as we can immediately perceive an improvement in the hearing. The contribution made by the pinna is one of the advantages of having a small hearing aid inside the canal rather than one placed behind the ear.

Animals with bigger ears have a clear advantage as they have muscles that prick up the ears automatically and point them in the right direction. Although these muscles are still present in humans they are only vestiges of the past and appear to have no function.

I had done a great deal of work recording the electrical responses to sound from these muscles as that can tell us if a newly born baby can hear. I felt very flattered when, at a medical gathering, I was told that a well-known physician was very anxious to meet me and had kept asking when I was coming. I was brought to him right away and his face lit up with delight.

"At last you are here!" he said, taking me aside. "I want to show you something."

He wanted me to look at his rather large ears and began to waggle them furiously. He was only satisfied when I admitted I had never seen anyone able to do this so well.

Of course not everyone is proud of having large ears and there is quite a demand for cosmetic surgery to correct "bat ears". I have not found any measurable difference in the actual ability to hear after the operation.

The ear canal itself is about two and a half centimetres long but is S-shaped rather than straight. It is lined with skin and at its bottom is the eardrum. By pulling the pinna upwards and outwards we can often see the drum reflecting the light. This is particularly easy to do in small children.

At one time some people believed that they could learn a lot from the shape of the ear including criminality. Recently I read that we can deduce the likelihood of heart disease from the appearance of the ear lobes but I am not convinced by either belief.

2.1.2.2 *The middle ear*

The eardrum or tympanic membrane separates the canal, which ends blindly at that point, from the cavity of the middle ear. As the canal is a cul-de-sac made of skin, its thin bottom layer is the outer surface of the drum.

The inner layer, on the other hand, is the continuation of the lining of the respiratory system. This continuous sheet of cells produces mucus so that, unlike skin, its surface is moist. The inner layer lines the Eustachian tube and covers the whole interior surface of the middle ear cavity and the drum. Because of its mucus-secreting properties it is called a *mucus membrane*. It developed, of course, from the first pouch that grows out of the inner tube or gut of the embryo.

There is a third layer between the skin and the mucus membrane which belongs exclusively to the tympanic membrane. It consists of strong fibres radiating towards the centre from a ring around the rim which hold it taut like the membrane of a drum.

There is a problem here with nomenclature. One of my professors held that a drum consists of the whole instrument and not just its membrane and that when dealing with the ear we should by analogy call it either the "drum head" or the "tympanic membrane". I was impressed with this argument until defeated by common usage. In the end I accepted that language shifts and alters and that what is correct today may have been yesterday's slang and may yet become tomorrow's archaism. My original firmness was strengthened at first by the French, who do not call it "*le tambour*", but when I realised that the Arabs refer to it as "*al tabla*", also a musical instrument, I gave in.

The tympanic membrane or eardrum ends up as a disc, almost a circle, although perhaps more an ellipse about 9 mm in diameter which makes it about half the size of a 5p coin or of an American dime. It is strong and taught because of the fibres of the middle layer, but very thin, since the other two layers are only a single cell thick. The middle layer is not quite complete, however, as there is a gap at the top. This anatomical quirk can lead to untold anguish and tragedy when infection pushes in from there.

Remnants of the cartilage which had formed the first and second arches in the foetus have become three separate little bones or *ossicles* which articulate with one another. These are called the *malleus* or hammer, the *incus* or anvil and the *stapes* or stirrup. They were given these names by imaginative anatomists of the past because of their fancied resemblance to these implements. Some of these are obviously anachronistic as the anatomists named the bones according to objects familiar in their own time:

although everyone still has a hammer, few know what an anvil or stirrup look like and they may as well be referred to by their Latin names.

The malleus is attached to the tympanic membrane so that when the membrane vibrates in response to sound, the malleus does so too, its movement being like that of a little hammer.

It does not actually strike the incus as a hammer does the anvil, but it does transmit sound vibrations to it and this in turn sets the third ossicle, the stapes, in motion.

The stapes is the smallest bone in the body and it truly looks like a tiny stirrup. Its footplate is oval and lies in an opening of the same shape in the bony wall of the inner ear which we therefore call the *oval window*. When the footplate of the stapes moves in and out with sound vibrations, the vibrations are transmitted to the salty fluids that fill the chambers of the inner ear.

This series of tiny bones is called the *ossicular chain* and it acts as a system of levers. The area of the tympanic membrane is 14 times that of the oval window so that the effect of the leverage increases the force of the sound vibrations a great deal from the one to the other.

This vast increase in force is important because the sound vibrations have to hop from the air in the canal to the fluids of the inner ear. Anyone who has tried to call a child who is swimming under water will have discovered how this passage diminishes the force of the sound.

The middle ear, then, is a cavity closed off on one side by the drum. At its other end it communicates with the outside by the Eustachian tube which opens at the back of the nose. Its importance lies in making sure that the middle ear is always full of air. The ossicular chain transmits the sound vibrations from the drum to the inner ear and increases their intensity.

The seventh cranial nerve, known as the facial nerve as it supplies the muscles of the face, which not only allow us to smile and whistle but also to drink without dribbling, passes across the middle ear though it has nothing to do with hearing. This nerve looms dangerously large as it can be damaged during operations on the ear and if this happens that side of the face is paralysed.

Yet another nerve crosses the drum. This one is tiny and carries a few taste fibres from the tongue. It is called the *corda tympani* and is often damaged by disease and it is also frequently necessary to cut it during operations, which rarely causes complications.

2.1.2.3 *The inner ear*

Early anatomists identified the tiny structures of the inner ear and saw that it consists of a complicated system of passages leading from one small cavity to another.

They could just about discern, lying in three planes, minute semicircular canals emerging from the little cavities. Cut across, the whole thing looks like a minuscule maze and so they called it the *labyrinth*, its Greek name. It is where our organ of balance is housed.

The hearing organ lies inside yet another of these channels that is coiled two and a half turns and we therefore call it the *cochlea,* which in Latin means snail shell.

We understand vibrations well enough. We can even imagine the ossicles of the middle ear moving back and forth, in response to the sound oscillations that have set the eardrum in motion, transmitting them to the fluids inside the labyrinthine cavities of the inner ear. We can accept also that waves corresponding to those of the original sounds in the air around us will be set up in these fluids.

What happens after that is still largely a mystery which our efforts have not completely resolved as although the known facts are many our understanding of what they mean is mainly theory and speculation.

How do ripples in the fluids of the inner ear, liquids which recall the primordial ocean from which all animals emerged, turn into the rich sounds that we perceive, into words and language, into the rhythms of poetry and the intricate harmonics of music?

The first step is more or less clear as we are dealing with sense organs we call *mechanoreceptors*. They are present all over the body and in their simplest form consist of a cell with a hair-like extension. The other end of the cell also projects outward but this time it forms a long thin fibre which, after passing through junctions and relay stations, ends up in the brain. This, of course brings to mind the *lateral line* in the primitive fish from which it may well have evolved.

We call such a collection of fibres bundled together a *sensory nerve* because it carries the sensation, whatever it happens to be, from each sensory organ but the real mystery is what takes place in the brain.

If the hair is tweaked, something happens to its cell. The mechanical movement gives rise to an electrical change which is then propagated along its fibre till it reaches the brain where, of course, the elusive seat of awareness lies.

That is straightforward enough and we can accept that if the vibrations are very vigorous the current induced might be very strong and that the appropriate functions of the brain will interpret it as very loud.

A greater problem is pitch. How is the pitch of a tone turned into an electric current that can be interpreted in the mind as the original tone?

One might expect that the rate of the vibrations decides the rate of the electrical impulses and that indicates the frequency of the tone. Experiments have shown that this actually happens only for the lower frequencies, as the rate of electrical impulses cannot keep up with that of the faster sound vibrations.

There must be some other way, perhaps like a keyboard, where the cells along the cochlea are responsible for the different frequencies according to which it is struck. The problem is where is the pianist that strikes them?

2.1.2.4 *Where is the pianist?*

When I was a junior doctor I was sent to collect a Nobel Prize-winner from London Heathrow Airport. I was to take him directly to where he was giving a lecture and although I was only the chauffeur I took it as a considerable honour.

Georg von Békésy was Hungarian but he had lived for many years in the United States. The first thing he did when I introduced myself was to ask if I spoke French. When I said that it was my first language he seemed relieved. As one grew older, he explained, the layers of memory peel away leaving us with the bare framework of our minds and as they had spoken French in his family in Budapest that was where he remained most comfortable. He suggested that it would be my fate too in due course.

He had put forward the theory of a travelling wave. Along the length of the cochlea there stretches a membrane called the *basilar membrane*, a sheet that carries some 17,000 hair cells, which form the sensory part of the hearing organ. This organ is called the Organ of Corti after the Italian anatomist who first described it properly. It is the cells at one end of that membrane that respond to the higher frequencies and those at the tip which respond to the lower pitches.

Von Békésy had suggested that the sound vibrations entering the inner ear at one end shook the membrane producing ripples along it but as each ripple advanced according to its frequency it was the place where it was displaced or shaken most that decided the pitch (Figure 5).

I had not understood it clearly when I had read his work, which was full of mathematical calculation as he had been trained as a telephone engineer. He explained it again at my request as I drove him into London, I think because he was so relieved to be able to speak French.

Perhaps it was the language of my childhood that took me back in time, but in listening to him my memories placed me on the roof of our building in Cairo where the washing was done and then put out to dry in the bright sunshine and unpolluted air of the time. The folding of the bed sheets, now gleaming white with the softness of the Egyptian cotton was a favourite

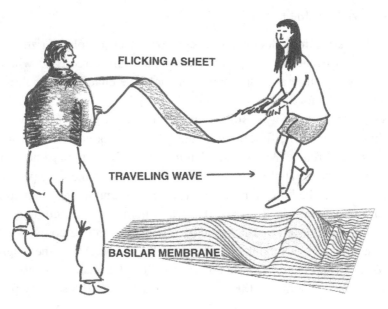

Figure 5. Travelling wave on the basilar membrane of the cochlea.

moment. Om Labib, the washerwoman would hold one end of the sheet and my nanny the other. They would tug this way and that to pull it taut, and then bring the two ends together to fold it.

I would beg them to let me hold one of the sheet and they often did so, even though they knew what I would do. As we pulled it taut I would flick my end and this would create a wave along the sheet which I watched with delight as it reached my nanny at the other end and jerked it out of her hands. That wave was the travelling wave and I understood it with the memory of childhood in the heat of the sun.

I still do not know where Professor von Békésy first got the idea that won him the Nobel Prize. Maybe it simply entered his mind from his knowledge of mathematics, but from what he told me I got the impression that he too may have come to that conclusion from similar uncomplicated childhood images. The part of the membrane that is the most severely displaced, like that of the sheet, depends on the length of the wave and that is the pitch we hear.

The electrical impulses emerging from the cells of the basilar membrane selected for their different frequencies, in their different fibres insulated from each other by their sheaths of myelin, are bundled together as the nerve of hearing, the eighth cranial nerve. This nerve now enters the skull through an opening to reach the brain.

2.1.2.5 Perception

The middle ear intensifies the sound vibrations it receives from the outer ear by means of the ossicular chain and transmits them through the oval window. The inner ear changes the sound vibrations into electrical impulses according to a code which we know only imperfectly but which is important if we are to improve cochlear implants and hearing aids.

The code indicates the loudness and the complex interplay of frequencies that result in what we hear. It is in this form that the sounds of the world about us, whether in the shape of speech, of music or only as background noise, reach a part of the brain called the *temporal lobe*.

It is in the superficial part of the cortex or outer layer of this lobe that awareness of sounds resides, as damage makes it difficult to sort them out into meaningful impressions even if the ear itself is intact.

I would have liked to know exactly the mechanism by which the world of sound, encoded into electrical impulses, takes the psychological form of awareness, interpretation and understanding. I would have liked to know in what way this is checked with the memory of sounds previously heard, and where this database, as we would call it now, resides. We learn a little bit more each day but we still do not have enough.

2.1.2.6 Balance

The organ of balance, the labyrinth, shares the same convoluted cavity and is bathed in the same fluids as the organ of hearing, the cochlea. It is also called the *vestibule* or *vestibular system*, which comes from the Latin for entrance hall.

The balance organ is similar to that of hearing as the sensory cells are also hair cells, and it is the mechanical bending of those structures which sets off an electrical impulse in the nerve of balance, the vestibular nerve.

The semicircular canals are in three planes, and when we move forwards, backwards or sideways, the resulting flow of the fluids inside them bends the hair cells indicating the direction in which we are going. The cavities from which the canals emerge also have hair cells but these carry little crystals stuck to their surface. Even when we are still, these minute stones pull the hair structure down because of gravity and that is the indication of our position relative to the ground.

No wonder astronauts in an environment free from gravity have problems with balance!

The nerve of balance enters the skull on its way to the brain together with the nerve of hearing and the facial nerve which decides the movements of the face. Damage which affects one may well affect the others.

There are of course other senses which help us keep our balance together with the labyrinth. Vision is one, as even if the vestibular system is destroyed completely we can still see where we are. Another is called the *proprioceptive sense*, a word which is related to awareness of oneself. We have tiny organs which are sensitive to pressure in our muscles and joints as well as the skin and they too let us know the position of our limbs.

2.2 Measuring Hearing

The hearing level is the loudness of a sound that can just be perceived. Deafness is expressed as how much *loss* there is relative to normal hearing. Deafness varies with pitch so it is measured separately for a number of frequencies.

Being able to follow speech is not the same as just hearing the sounds.

The earliest test for deafness is:

"Can you hear me?"

If the subject is willing and able to cooperate, a series of tests based on that question or its refinements have been devised and are called *subjective tests*.

Sometimes a subject cannot or will not respond, as in the case of a baby or of a malingerer. Tests have been designed which observe the response and can be referred to as *objective tests*.

2.2.1 *Subjective tests*

The following are most commonly used:

- Voice
- Tuning fork tests
- Pure tone audiometry
- The loudness discomfort level
- Speech audiometry
- Automatic audiometry

2.2.1.1 *Voice*

The simplest way is "Can you hear what I am saying?" and "Can you hear me if I whisper?"

We can even quantify it a little by moving further away and asking "Can you still hear me?" and noting down the distance at which the subject can still hear.

That is what we did during my National Service as an Army doctor. We recited a standard list of words and the soldier was supposed to repeat what we said as we moved further away. It was recorded simply as:

CV (Conversational Voice): 15 ft

WV (Whispered Voice): 10 ft

This was not unreasonable for finding out whether a soldier could hear a command, but it was inadequate in two major ways. In the first place some speak softly while others tend to shout so the loudness is hardly standard. The second problem is to do with being understood. I became aware of the problem as soon as I arrived to do my clinic on my first day in the Army. The very first patient stood at attention, staring ahead.

"Sayrrheed!" he said.

"Sore head!" the sergeant translated and I wrote down "headache".

I had been sent to a Highland regiment in Scotland, and my standard English confused the young Glaswegian recruit. Words have to be understood as well as heard.

2.2.1.2 *Tuning forks*

The Army had provided me with an array of tuning forks of different frequencies. The sergeant, a pharmacist in civilian life, had been surprised as to what I was going to do. Were we going to play music?

If a tuning fork vibrating at 512 Hz (middle C) is pressed on to the top of the head, the vibrations will be transmitted directly to the inner ear through the skull, bypassing the outer and middle ears. If the hearing is normal the tone will be heard equally in both ears. It will sound "in the head".

If the inner ear or nerve do not function normally in one ear then it stands to reason that it will not be heard so well on the deaf side.

If the obstacle to hearing is in the outer or middle ear, it will seem louder on the deaf side! That means the nerve must be in good order and the deafness is due to a fault in the conduction mechanism. We call it *conductive deafness;* in Europe it is called *transmission deafness*. Both are good names and it means a great deal, as that type of deafness is often curable.

Patients may be surprised and amused, although some cannot believe, to know they are hearing the tuning fork better on their deaf side. Some overlook the evidence of their own senses.

No one has a problem comparing the loudness of the tuning fork when it is first presented in front of the ear and then pressed against the bone behind. Of course we can hear better through the ear otherwise we would not bother to have one. If we hear better on the bone it confirms that there is a blockage somewhere in the outer or middle ear, signifying that the deafness is *conductive* and hopefully curable. This test is called the Rinne test, named after the German otologist Heinrich Rinne.

2.2.1.3 *Pure tone audiometry*

For a more accurate test, we need to quantify hearing levels rather better than by merely saying "Can you hear me now?" and using tuning forks. We need decibels and Hertz.

The solution is the electrical *pure tone audiometer*.

It is now the standard method to test hearing and the record made using the audiometer is called an *audiogram*, although there has been a linguistic rebellion by some who insisted it should be an *audiograph*. The latter has not been widely taken up and I think it is a moot point, just like the *drum-head* vs *eardrum* argument.

The aim is to test the hearing for a number of separate pure tones. The frequencies chosen lie between 125 Hz and 8,000 Hz as that is the range most important for speech.

The subject puts on a pair of earphones and each ear is tested in turn.

The audiometer emits a tone when the tester presses a button and the patient gives a sign whenever he hears it. The frequencies commonly tested are:

250 Hz 500 Hz 1,000 Hz (1 kHz) 2 kHz 4 kHz 8 kHz

The aim is to find out the patient's hearing threshold and the extent of his or her deafness, if present. To this end we have a standard minimum audible level representing those of us who claim to be able to hear perfectly well.

Such a standard was set a long time ago by measuring in decibels the faintest sound that could just be heard by a large number of normally hearing people. This was done for the different frequencies separately and can be referred to as "normal hearing" or "0 dB of hearing loss" as there is no hearing loss (Figure 6).

If someone does have hearing loss the tone being tested must be made louder until he can just hear it. That is the value recorded in decibels.

The result is a chart, the pure tone audiogram. And as the tones have been transmitted through earphones producing sound vibrations in the air of the ear canal we call it more specifically an *air conduction (AC) audiogram.*

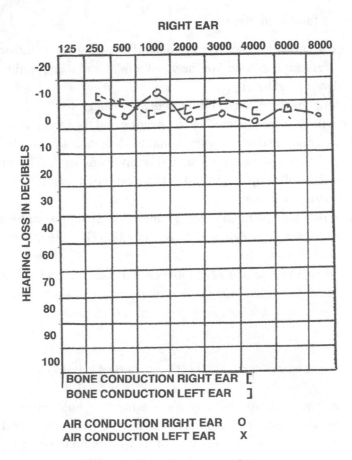

Figure 6. Normal pure tone audiogram.

Sound can also be transmitted directly through the skull by applying a vibrator tightly on the bone behind the ear, as with the tuning fork. The test is repeated in exactly the same way but with the vibrator and the graph. The results of this is called a *bone conduction (BC) audiogram.*

The reason for doing the test both ways is that if someone can hear better through the bone than by air conduction it means that there is an obstruction in the outer or middle ear. The inner ear and the nerve are intact since they can respond to vibrations if applied directly. As with the tuning fork test, the implications are enormous as the diagnosis and treatment depends on where the obstruction is.

To avoid misleading recordings, when the tone played to one ear is heard by the other, usually better, ear we make a masking sound in the ear that is not being tested.

Audiometry is done in a quiet room or, even better, in a soundproof booth.

2.2.1.4 *The loudness discomfort level*

Many people with a hearing aid complain that the "noise is too loud" even though the words they want to hear are not clear enough. Some suffering from certain conditions of the inner ear find that although they are deaf they are also singularly disturbed by loud sounds. The paradox of sounds being either not loud enough or too loud is difficult to live with.

This can be demonstrated with the audiometer in a simple manner by measuring the sound level at which they begin to feel uncomfortable. This level may be different for different tones.

If a normally hearing person listens through the earphones he will generally find 90 dB uncomfortably loud. A deaf person may require this degree of amplification simply in order to hear something but many suffer from a phenomenon we call *recruitment* and their discomfort level may be as low as 85 dB or even 80 dB. Here is where the paradox lies. We say they have a *narrow dynamic range.*

They are likely to have a serious problem with their hearing aids.

2.2.1.5 *Speech audiometry*

When a person complains that he is deaf he usually means that he cannot hear what people are saying. Of course there are many other problems like not being able to hear the traffic or an alarm, but the main disability is the difficulty with communication.

The speech audiogram is an attempt to demonstrate the problem.

A previously recorded list of standard words can be heard through earphones so the test can be performed for each ear separately. It can also be done in a quiet room or soundproof booth using a loudspeaker listening with both ears and even while wearing a hearing aid.

The patient tries to recognise lists of words which have been balanced to include all the frequencies of speech at different intensities and the percentage of correctly identified words is plotted against the loudness.

This is useful when checking hearing aids but it is very time-consuming and the information obtained is not particularly helpful other than in testing the value of hearing aids.

2.2.1.6 *Automatic audiometry*

Von Békésy devised a test that is mainly self-administered and has therefore been useful in an industrial setting where a large number of people need to be tested.

The subject puts on earphones and a continuous tone is heard in each ear at a time. The tone goes from a range of low pitches to high pitches.

Its loudness is controlled by the patient who presses a button when the sound gets so faint that he cannot hear. This switches it on again so he lets go until the sound gets fainter again.

The graph which results is not very accurate but it is useful as a screening test.

2.2.2 **Objective tests**

We started working on electrical responses to sound in the hope that we might make a machine that would show us whether a small child, at birth even, could hear or not. Our requirements were that there would be little room for error and for people with little training to be able to do the test correctly.

We wanted to know if a baby could hear when we had realised that early detection and intervention made an important difference to the outcome regarding speech and language development, but we were also aware that half the children with a hearing loss were not identified until it was obvious from the fact that they could not speak.

Maybe we were wrong to call them "objective tests" as it caused a philosophical controversy.

"If I clap my hands and the child blinks," a sceptic said, "that is an objective enough sign that it hears. You have to check that the graph in your electrical test is not just static or something. You still have to decide."

There is no such argument today and when our patient cannot or will not cooperate we use a number of techniques that fall into three groups of tests:

- A sound evokes an electrical response in the brain.
- We measure sounds emitted by the cochlea: otoacoustic emissions
- We measure the mechanical functions of the middle ear: tympanometry

2.2.2.1 *Electrical responses*

The Franco-Prussian War of 1870 was one of those events by which we trace the later course of history. Napoleon III abdicated and went to live in Cheltenham, and Germany became an imperial power ready to enter into a world war. It was a time when the scientific interest of the Enlightenment received the technological tools of the 19th century. However, of particular interest to us is the fact that on that fateful battle-field a physician is said to have recorded electrical changes with an electrode placed directly on the brain of a soldier who had had the top of his skull shot off.

Sixty years later, Hans Berger of Jena, in Prussia, recorded the brain's electrical responses with electrodes placed on the scalp and our own work evolved from there. Hearing sounds caused changes in the electrical patterns of the brain but they were too small and erratic to use as an indication of hearing until computers came.

Hearing a tone causes a tiny electrical wave indistinguishable from the other squiggles resulting from the brain's activity but it can be repeated endless times, the minute responses stacked into a visible spike by the computer, while the responses to other external or internal stimuli — the

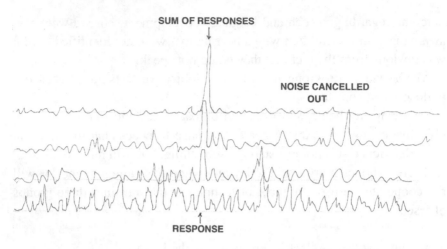

Figure 7. An electrical response adds up to become visible

other squiggles on the screen — appear randomly and do not increase in size despite repetition, cancelling each other out. As the sounds are repeated many times the responses to them add up, becoming more obvious (Figure 7).

True hearing levels can be obtained when people are feigning deafness but we cannot rely on electrical responses from the brain in small children as it is necessary for the patient to keep very still for a long time; putting them to sleep cancels the responses.

I struggled with the question of how to overcome the problem of collecting responses to sound from a small, wriggling child. One day I was sitting on Hampstead Heath thinking about the problem while watching people walk their dogs. One creature sat, looking intent, when there was a faint, almost imperceptible sound in the grass. The dog instantly pricked up its ears and, as a result, put an idea in my mind.

Placing electrodes behind my own ears I saw responses swamp the computer screen when the speakers sounded even faint clicks. They had come from the muscles behind my ears, normally a nuisance to researchers, being too variable themselves to be used as an indicator of hearing.

Pricking up the ears, a response to quiet sounds was what we had been looking for and although our ears may not move in the same way as a dog's, they try to, and the electrical signals that resulted were the efforts of my weak vestigial muscles.

Head movements altered these electrical responses making them unreliable but by recording from both sides at once and by getting our computer to add them up we obtained a recording which we called the *crossed acoustic response*.

It served us well for some years to help identify many children who were deaf at birth or a young age, although it has since been replaced by even more reliable methods.

2.2.2.2 *Auditory brainstem responses (ABR)*

One day a slight, diffident man came to visit us from Jerusalem. Professor Moshe Feinmesser wanted to show us something he and his colleague, Haim Sohmer, had found. Rearranging our recording equipment, he placed an electrode on the top of his head where it stuck easily as he was bald.

After the usual series of clicks, the screen showed a response we had not seen before (Figure 8). Little dips and bumps appeared, each representing a step in the path taken by the electrical impulse evoked by the sound, from the inner ear to the brain though not as far as the areas where we perceive and understand.

It is Sohmer and Feinmesser's work that resulted in the auditory brainstem response (ABR) test, currently used in testing babies today. It has been automated, which means it can be carried out by non-specialists as a screening test all over the world

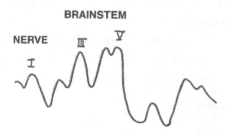

Figure 8. Brain stem responses.

2.2.2.3 *Otoacoustic emissions*

In the late 1970s I was told that a young researcher, David Kemp, had made a remarkable discovery and I went to seek him out as he was working down the road in London.

In fact he was not easy to find as I had to make my way down the narrow steps of the old Royal National Nose Throat and Ear Hospital at the top end of Gray's Inn Road, near King's Cross Station.

When I reached the basement I wandered down dark corridors to David Kemp's gloomy little laboratory but what he showed me, was quite extraordinary. He had found, by placing a microphone in the ear, that the ear *produces* sounds.

It is know that the ear responds to sound, but that it actually *emits* sounds seemed, to say the least, improbable. Many disregarded the observation that did not conform to the expected, but Kemp persisted and we now know that the cochlea emits acoustic energy, but only if it is functioning normally.

I was so excited that I telephoned Dr Abraham Shulman, a professor of ear, nose and throat at the SUNY/Downstate University who had organised a world conference on hearing and tinnitus in New York. I told him he must invite this man, pay his fare, his hotel, whatever was necessary, as he had a rare new discovery to show us.

These unexpected sounds, actually made by the normal ear, were called *otoacoustic emissions* and turned out to be a good indication of the hearing level. Because of the rapidity and ease with which the sounds could be measured, they proved to be ideal for babies, so much so that, in 1993, when the United States National Institutes of Health held a consensus conference and called for a national screening programme of the newborn, they recommended this test as a standard. I find it curious that it was introduced only two years later in the United Kingdom and the NHS newborn screening programme as we know it did not get under way until 2002.

2.2.2.4 *Tympanometry*

This is a completely different type of test as it does not measure electrical responses to sound. It measures the movement of the drum, which allows

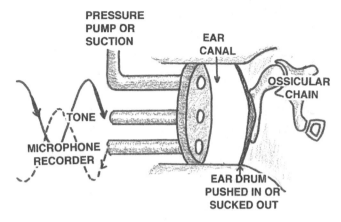

Figure 9. Tympanometer.

us to deduce what the air pressure is in the middle ear as well as how well the Eustachian tube is functioning.

It does all that in a very ingenious manner: An airtight plug pierced by three tubes is placed in the ear canal. The first tube emits a tone which is reflected on the surface of the drum. The reflected sound wave, which returns through the second tube, cancels out the outgoing one (Figure 9).

The third tube is connected to a pump which can suck air out of the canal or pump it in. If it is airtight the pressure sucks the eardrum outwards or pushes it in so that when it moves, the reflected wave will be displaced. The movement is indicated on a graph.

If the pressure in the middle ear is normal and the air can pass in and out of the Eustachian tube without hindrance, the graph will show a sharp peak when the pressure in the canal is the same as that in the middle ear.

If the Eustachian tube is not functioning well, for instance when we have a cold, the peak will be smaller and displaced to the negative side.

If the middle ear is filled with fluid, such as happens with "glue ear" there will be no peak at all and the graph will be flat (Figure 10).

Tympanometry will also give us information about the ossicular chain. When the ossicular chain is stiff as a result of disease, the pressure may be normal but the peak will be less sharp and very small. If, on the contrary, the chain has been interrupted, the drum will be looser and the peak relatively higher.

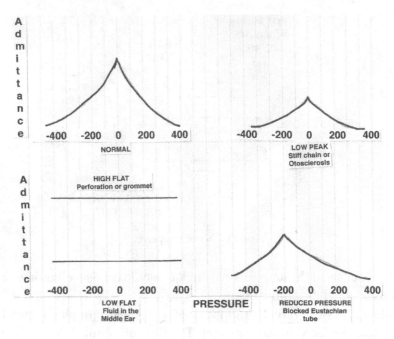

Figure 10. Tympanometry responses.

These measurements, however, do not tell us if the ear can hear, but it is able to measure a tiny reflex. The stapes may be the smallest bone in the body but attached to it is an even smaller muscle, the *stapedius*. This muscle helps to protect the cochlea from loud noises by holding on tightly to the bone to prevent it from vibrating too intensely. Although it is not very effective in that role, the little movement made by the stapedius can be detected by the tympanometer and gives an indication that something was heard.

2.3 Names and Nomenclature

Eustachian tube, Organ of Corti and so on are named after important scientists. But who were these people? Do we need these names? I suppose not, but these names have stuck, while I have changed my views more than once.

I had strong opinions when I was a junior doctor and believed, for instance, that it was wrong to call the inner ear both the *labyrinth* and the *vestibular system* as one was Greek and the other Latin. My consultant at the time kept on about the tympanic membrane being the *drumhead* rather than the *eardrum*, but it was the Eustachian tube that led me to take a less pedantic view.

There was a sort of iconoclastic movement in the 1960s, perhaps the same one that disapproved of putting statues on pedestals, that wanted to get rid of eponymous names such as Parkinson's disease or Hodgkin's disease. The first, they felt should be *hyperkinetic rigid syndrome* and the second should have been *Reed–Sternberg lymphoma* except that they did not want to perpetuate Dr Reed or Dr Sternberg either. They tried to change the *Eustachian tube* to the *nasopharyngeal tube* but it did not take on with patients as, although "Eustachian" was difficult to pronounce or spell, "nasopharyngeal" sounded more like a serious disease than the familiar tube we try to unblock when we have a cold or are in an airplane.

Bartolomeo Eustachi, an Italian anatomist from the 16th century deserves some remembrance by people concerned with the ear as his was the first correct description of its anatomy. Yet the Church prevented the publication of his book *Anatomical Engravings* until more than 100 years after his death. Why they did this is and why they were so worried about it is not entirely clear even now.

Alphonse Giacomo Gaspare Corti's was quite a different story as he lived in an enlightened 19th century Italy. He was the Marquess of Santo Stefano Belbo while his younger brother was the Foreign Minister of the new kingdom of Italy. In 1851 he described the anatomy of the spiral-shaped sensory organ of hearing in the cochlea and it has been known ever since as the Organ of Corti. This was a most important achievement and his original histological preparations are still kept in the Anatomical Museum in Vienna, where he had qualified in medicine.

As for muscles and electrical impulses, it was not I who discovered them but Luigi Galvani who taught at the University of Bologna in the late 18th century. He had called it *bioelectricity* and when I was working on the electrical response to sound in the vestigial muscles behind the ear, I became interested in him. His was a well-ordered life: he held the Chair of Natural Science at Bologna which, interestingly, in those days was still called "Natural Magic" and was happily married to the accomplished and attractive daughter of a fellow professor. He reached respected retirement but history did not let him rest as, when Napoleon invaded Italy, Galvani refused to swear allegiance to the new Cisalpine Republic and his pension was withdrawn. Presumably Napoleon had not been impressed by his work on bioelectricity even though his book had been a bestseller. When the Emperor had been defeated, however, Galvani's pension was restored with compensation, although he had died by then.

Interestingly, Mary Wollstonecraft (or Mary Shelley, as she is better known, after she married Percy Shelley) had read his book on a holiday at the Villa Diodati near Lake Geneva with Percy Shelley, Lord Byron and the physician John Polidori. It rained most of the time and the party decided they would each write a horror story. Wollstonecraft, full of Galvani's experiments on making dead or disembodied muscles twitch and seemingly come to life, invented Dr Frankenstein and his monster. Polidori in turn wrote one of the first vampire stories in his short story *The Vampyre*.

Heinrich Adolph Rinne developed his eponymous test to distinguish between two types of deafness. He has become a familiar name in the medical world by the frequent use of the terms "Rinne positive" and Rinne negative". He was a doctor in Göttingen, Germany and a contemporary of Corti. He received no credit for his test, which has become perhaps the most-used test in otological practice, as it only became popular after his death.

Hans Berger's is yet another story as, after the Second World War, the German Society of Neurophysiology instituted a Hans Berger triennial prize to celebrate his work on the electrical responses of the brain but recent research has shown that his diaries are full of anti-Semitic remarks. On retirement he had been appointed to the Court of Genetic Health set up by the Nazis and was thus responsible for deciding who was to be sterilised. It is not possible to know now what turbulence went on in his mind as he hanged himself in 1941.

2.4 Testing Children

When I joined Guy's Hospital I took over what was known as the "Deaf Children's Clinic".

The name was inappropriate as, though there was no lack of patients, they were all children who had failed to develop speech. Some were indeed deaf, but many had other developmental problems which I was unable to handle by myself, whether they had hearing loss or not.

I asked the Newcomen Centre, a department set up at Guy's to look after children with developmental disorders, for help. It was itself a relatively recent speciality, although the neurological evaluation of children as a separate entity had existed at the Hôpital Sainte Anne in Paris since 1940.

I changed the name of my clinic to the Hearing and Language Clinic, and Dr Dorothy Egan, a developmental paediatrician, agreed to join me. We invited a teacher of the deaf, Pamela Snowden, who had been trained in Manchester by Professor Sir Alexander Ewing and his wife, Ethel. The Ewings, very influential in their time, insisted that oral training exclude visual clues. Indeed, Pamela had had her hand slapped by Lady Ewing after unwittingly using a gesture while talking to a deaf child. A speech therapist, Yasmin Saklatwallah, joined us too, and so we examined our young patients together and our clinic at the Newcomen Centre was a template for the way the assessment of children evolved in the United Kingdom.

A child is a constantly moving target, as what we have to assess is in the process of development, and changes day by day. Indeed, the rate of change itself is what we measure.

Testing the hearing of older children can be done as that of adults but in the case of young ones our approach has to be different.

A young child does not complain of hearing loss. It may be that the parents are suspicious because of an early lack of response to sounds or a delay in developing speech. A school-age child may sit looking out of the window oblivious to what the teacher is saying. Poor performance may be the only indication that the hearing is not adequate.

If deafness is not recognised early, it may deprive the baby of the opportunity to learn how to speak at all. In school-age children, education and life prospects may be blighted by even a mild hearing loss.

We design our tests not only to detect the presence of hearing loss, but also to differentiate the profoundly deaf from those that are moderately or mildly affected. Hearing is often impaired only for certain frequencies such as the higher tones. Other children have a fluctuating hearing loss and may be entirely normal if examined during the warm months of the summer holidays but can hardly hear during the recurrent colds of winter.

These special problems have led to a dual approach in the assessment of children's hearing. Testing is done both in response to parental doubt or teachers' suspicion and by screening all children at different stages in their development.

Governments, often under pressure from the public, have set up screening programmes when there have not been sufficient trained personnel available. Mistakes then are doubly dangerous as they may give a false sense of security or lead to unnecessary intervention.

When no arrangements have been made to deal with the outcome, there have also been disastrous results. At one time I discovered that the findings of screening tests for hearing loss in school age children had simply been filed away in the archives of the Inner London Education Authority.

2.4.1 *Screening for hearing loss*

Screening is relatively recent in medicine and has already become controversial. In some ways it is a social project if not also a philosophical one and, as it involves public expense, it borders on the political as well as on economics. One question that arises is whether we screen every single child (universal screening) or concentrate on those with risk factors. Ideally, though, both screenings should be done, as 40% of deaf children do not seem to have any known risk factor. Today our societies are demographically very fluid with much external and internal migration, making it easy for children to miss out if they happen not to be there that day or if the parents fear drawing attention to themselves. Hearing loss may develop later and some limited frequency loss can be missed by the tests.

In the United Kingdom, until 2006 when the screening programme involved behavioural tests at 9 months and 18 months, it was clear that half of those with hearing loss had been missed while a quarter had still to be identified by two and a half years or even three years. On the NHS today, the first screening test is carried out in the maternity ward before discharge or at home by a health visitor. The aim is for all babies to be screened within the first few weeks of life. The test used is the automated otoacoustic emission (AOAE) test which takes a few minutes and is done best while the baby is asleep.

Unless there is a clear result in both ears the test is repeated soon after in a quieter environment. If necessary an ABR or an automated ABR is carried out, and if there appears to be hearing loss, the screen is followed up by referral to the audiology clinic.

Whether we should have an audiogram as a screening test when children enter school is more controversial. It is naturally a good thing to know whether a child is deaf, but as the main cause of hearing loss in that age group is "glue ear", and as that fluctuates between summer and winter, we may be falsely reassured by a good result.

2.4.2 *Follow up*

Follow up involves the history, observation and examination of the child's hearing and we need to know how the child responds to quiet sounds, not just loud ones.

A baby will suddenly keep very still if it hears its mother tiptoeing into a carpeted room and quite small children react very quickly to the sound of their father's key turning in the lock. However, if a child looks up when an airplane is passing overhead it only confirms that it can hear the low frequencies of engine's hum, though it may still be deaf to the high ones such as the sound "s" and "f". A deaf baby may not babble as much or in the same tones as one who hears normally. Older children may want to turn up the volume of the television.

The risk factors must be investigated. These include a family history of deafness and any evidence of perinatal infection. Rubella during pregnancy was once a major cause of foetal abnormality as well as deafness but it will hopefully disappear if the MMR vaccination programme continues to be applied. After birth it is meningitis, encephalitis and mumps that are significant.

Low birth weight babies have a higher risk of deafness, as well as those who have developed jaundice or who have been injured during labour. Babies who have received special care and have low Apgar scores are considered at risk. Although "Apgar" now serves as an acronym for assessing the health of newborn babies (Appearance, Pulse, Grimace, Activity, Respiration), it was originally named after Dr Virginia Apgar who introduced it at Columbia University in the United States.

2.4.3 *Observation and examination*

We obtain much valuable information by observing the child at any age especially when it does not feel watched. Talking to the parents often allows children to lose interest and if the hearing is normal mentioning their name will elicit a surreptitious look.

Physical examination includes the ears, nose and throat and a check for cranio-facial abnormalities and cleft palate as well as the eyes, heart and neurological systems and signs of developmental delay.

2.4.4 *Tests*

Our aim is to test the hearing for a range of frequencies from 500 Hz to 8,000 Hz as it includes the sounds used in speech. We also want to know that the child can hear sounds at least at 30 dB. Anything outside that range of pitch and loudness may later result in impaired speech in the baby and in educational failure in the school-age child.

The tests depend on whether the child is able to cooperate or not. Inability to cooperate may be because the child is too young but the cause may also be developmental delay. A child who has a mental age of two can only be tested as we would a two-year-old, even if it is much older.

2.4.4.1 *If the child cannot cooperate*

Even a very tiny baby will blink if we clap our hands loudly or shout "BA!" They may even show signs of distress so we know, at least, that it has heard that sound.

From the age of six months a baby has enough control of his head and neck muscles to turn to check where a sound is coming from.

As our aim is to make sure that most of the frequencies necessary for speech are heard it would be very helpful if our baby turned to each of the pure tones of the audiogram but they are not interesting enough and we have to use sounds that the baby would want to explore.

There is no sound more interesting than the human voice, even when the baby has no idea what we are saying. Useful sounds include: "sss" as that is a high frequency sound and "oo" as that is a low frequency sound. The baby's name, when whispered or spoken at a conversational volume, is also worthwhile for testing hearing, even in babies.

Food is naturally very interesting to babies and rubbing a spoon around the rim of a cup will make the baby turn to look. Many other sound sources have been used in this way but we must be sure that the sound we make is not loud. In the clinics we measure the sound we are making with a sound-level meter and if the baby can hear sounds of less than 30 dB the hearing is good enough to develop speech without special help.

These tests are called *distraction tests* as they involve distracting the baby but they have to be carefully controlled. I remember once when a visitor came to watch a test being carried out. She was decked out with brilliant jewellery and shiny necklaces. The babies could not keep their eyes off her and it was impossible to get them to turn away no matter how loud the sound.

The person who is making the sounds must be out of sight but babies can be very astute. Once, one of our testers was wearing a perfume which was apparently very attractive, so that the babies would turn around when she crept up behind them whether they could hear her or not.

Discovering the person who is making the sound is exciting for the baby and sufficient reward in itself, but not for long. By the age of 18 months the baby has lost interest in that simple game and a new test is needed.

Testing the hearing of a blind baby in this way is very difficult as we depend on it turning to see what has made the sound. If the baby cannot see anything it will not have learnt to turn. Many cases have been referred as suspected deafness because the child had failed to turn to a sound; in fact the child could hear perfectly well but was blind.

2.4.4.2 *When the child is beginning to cooperate*

This is when babies are more interested in handing over or pointing to familiar objects like a spoon, a cup, a toy car or airplane, a doll or a brush when asked: "Give me the ..."

By the age of two they will be able to point to parts of their body: "Show me your nose!"

We have to be careful that the child cannot see our lips move as those with a hearing loss become extremely good at visual clues from the eyes or facial expression.

After the age of two children are very interested in pictures as well as toys and they will point or play with them very happily. Toys that are too complex can sometimes be too absorbing for children as they may refuse to let go of it and lose interest in anything else.

By the age of three most children will place a brick in a box in response to a pure tone and soon after this age they can do this with the earphones on. The child is now performing a pure tone audiogram. Children are able and pleased to do this between the ages of three and four.

If the child is unable to cooperate by playing these games it may well be deaf but another reason may be that it is globally delayed and here is another instance of the need to understand how the child is performing as a whole rather than only in regard to its hearing. A general developmental assessment is essential in conjunction with specific hearing tests whether we are screening or responding to parental doubt.

2.4.4.3 *Objective tests*

AOAE and ABR are now used mainly as part of the screening process. When children are developing normally and show normal responses to sound at the right stages there is no need for electrical tests at all. People complain at times that their children had not been properly tested because "It was only someone who whispered behind her." Those who have a greater respect for technology then for observation will never be convinced.

If there is doubt, objective tests come into their own, particularly if the intellectual development of the child is impaired.

Part II

Deafness

It is traditional to divide deafness into two types, Conductive and Perceptive, now usually called Neurosensory. Balance and tinnitus cannot be separated from deafness.

We know what deafness is, but there is also degree to deafness, and how we respond to it. Those living alone, watching television in command of the loudness button, may feel they can hear well enough for their needs even if they are very deaf. Those who may have only a slight hearing loss but work in business and enjoy an active social life, may find that when talking to grandchildren or attending the theatre will complain they "cannot hear a thing!"

In the West, where disability of every sort including deafness from noise exposure generates special entitlements and where monetary compensation is available, there is a demand for a mathematical definition of deafness and its severity.

Organisations which previously described themselves as serving the deaf now often refer to the "deaf and hard of hearing" so it is necessary to include people who experience some difficulty as well, although it is difficult to know what numbers are involved.

It is said that in the United States there are more than 20 million people who have a hearing problem. The old European Union of 12 nations calculated that 1% of its citizens were deaf, which comes to 35 million; in the United Kingdom alone the Royal National Association of Deaf people claims to represent 9 million people on its website.

Whichever way the figures are worked out the numbers are large, and there are three broad causes: heredity, illness and environmental factors. The final cause varies but includes accidents, exposure to excessive noise and other hazards, some affecting the unborn.

The greatest single reason why hearing problems continue to increase is simply that we are an ageing population and our hearing fades as we get older.

I was once asked to test High Court judges and law Lords as many were elderly and had some hearing loss, but when I watched them at work I found that they were all coping very well.

On the other hand a barrister insisted that his career would end unless he was fitted with an aid, even though I told him that his hearing was certainly no worse than that of the judges.

"It is not the same," he said. "Everyone in court has to address the judge, who can tell the witnesses to speak up. For me it is a nightmare when I cannot see their lips."

Even a slight degree of hearing loss in only one ear can make life difficult for some people, while others, who may lead an entirely different life and have a different job, can manage with very little hearing.

Jack Ashley, the Labour peer, was profoundly deaf. He told me that the onset of deafness, sudden or slow, can be disastrous for a person: sudden deafness is traumatic; the slow development of deafness is insidious. Ultimately, he said, the results are the same: deafness results in loss of confidence, increasing misunderstanding, social isolation and, occasionally, demoralisation.

Some people consider deafness to be worse than blindness as it affects the ability to communicate by speech with one's fellows, to hear the tone of their voices, and to catch the barely perceptible modulations that tell us so much; these subtle nuances are harder to hide than facial expression.

Attitudes to deafness has varied over time but as it can strike every family, every age and every social class there has always been both compassion and concern for those afflicted. In the Bible, God's instruction to Moses sets the tone which most societies have, by and large, accepted:

"Speak unto all the congregation of the children of Israel and say unto them: 'Thou shalt not curse the deaf nor put an obstacle before the blind, but shalt fear thy God. I am the Lord'" (Leviticus 19:14).

On the other hand a large part of humour in most cultures relates to mis-understandings and deafness lends itself to this. Renoir in his film *Une Partie de Campagne* shamelessly poked fun at problems of communication, though today it may be considered an affront to the disabled.

Advances in understanding the nature of deafness have helped to reduce its effects, particularly in the second half of the 20th century. However, the first step was that made in 1855 by Heinrich Adolf Rinne, the general practitioner from Göttingen, when he demonstrated, by using a tuning fork, that there were two types of deafness: *conductive* and what was then known as *perceptive*.

The difference between the two is crucial, as conductive deafness can often be cured.

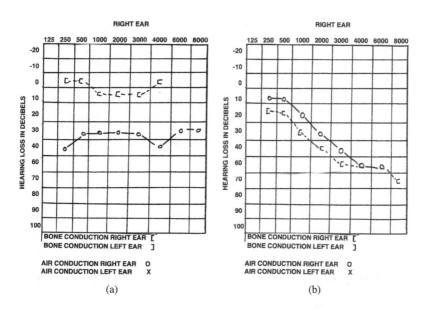

(a)   (b)

Figure 11. Audiogram showing (a) conductive (b) neurosensory hearing loss in the right ears of two different people.

Although we can tell the difference between conductive and perceptive deafness with a tuning fork as in the Rinne test, if we want a quantitative record we need to carry out a pure tone audiogram.

If the hearing loss is less when tested by bone conduction than by air conduction, that is, tones seem louder when pressed on the bone behind the ear, the deafness is conductive. If not, it is neurosensory (Figure 11).

Two other aspects that will be discussed in this part are loss of balance and tinnitus, which are closely related to deafness. Finally, deafness from birth is special as it impedes the development of speech.

Chapter 3

Conductive Deafness

The obstacle to the transmission of sound lies in the outer or the middle ear.

3.1 Disease of the Outer Ear

3.1.1 *Wax*

It is normal to have wax in the ears as it is produced by tiny glands in the skin of the canal in the same way that glands over the rest of the body produce sweat. In fact these wax-making structures are probably modified sweat glands.

Ear wax forms a protective coat over the thin skin. The wax is carried along to be shed at the opening of the ear-hole. Sometimes the ear wax is not shed and it accumulates, blocking the canal and causing deafness and frustration.

We do not always know why this happens, although in some instances it is obvious, for example blockages can result from excessive use of cotton wool buds in an attempt to clean the ears or to dry them after washing.

Swimming and especially diving can also push the wax deep into the canal. This means the hearing loss is immediate, as the water also gets absorbed by the wax. It may even be painful because of the pressure exerted by the swollen wax, which crushes the thin skin against the bone.

Eczema around the ear-hole can also act as a barrier, preventing wax getting out, often also causing irritation and the need to rub and scratch the ear. Scratching, especially with cotton wool buds, matches, or other tools, can only make things worse. It can, however, be kept under control with a cortisone cream.

If it cannot be prevented the obstructing wax must be removed by a practitioner.

I have heard that, in return for a small fee, street practitioners will do this for passers-by in India with a special little tool. I suppose everything is possible, but as these practitioners cannot possibly see what they are doing, such procedures are not entirely safe.

A few years ago a technique, said to be of Native American origin, gained popularity and praise from those who prefer natural cures to contemporary medication. The technique is called "candling" and it involves conducting the heat of a lighted candle through a tube inserted into the ear canal. I suspect the procedure melts the wax but its vogue seems to have diminished in this country. The procedure is relatively safe — I don't know of a case where anyone has got burned.

Traditionally, ears were syringed with water to wash out the wax and this is perfectly satisfactory but it requires some skill and it should not be done if there is an infection present or a perforation of the eardrum. In the past syringing had been a standard procedure for the general practitioner, after the patient used drops for a week or two to soften the wax beforehand, but it has now tended to fall into disfavour.

Specialists can sometimes pick out the wax with an instrument as they examine the ear, and there are few patients who are as delighted as those who are freed from the blockage. Because general practitioners and nurses are now less willing to syringe ears (largely due to increasing litigation associated with intervention), the use of drops to dissolve wax has become very popular. There are many commercial preparations, and though they are effective in the long run, the ear initially feels even deafer as the drops add to the sensation of blockage.

Ordinary sodium bicarbonate ear drops are harmless and can be obtained from the chemist without a prescription, but it is possible to develop a reaction to other chemicals. Olive oil and almond oil, although popular, are ineffective as solvents. Their use is to soften the wax sufficiently for the doctor or the nurse to syringe the ear more easily. It must be remembered that only experienced practitioners should remove wax from the ear using this method. Trying to remove the wax with cotton buds or other implements may cause damage. Softened wax can also be removed with an electric sucker, provided the wax is not too hard, but the procedure should be done by a specialist using a microscope.

Women who have had face lifts are now more frequent sufferers from blockage by wax as the skin has sometimes been pulled up past the ear canal narrowing to a slit which is easily obstructed.

3.1.2 *Infection in the canal*

Infection of the outer ear often happens as a result of swimming, which indicates that these organisms must be floating about in pools despite efforts at disinfection. I used to think that the sea was safe until I attended a seminar on outer ear infections from swimming and what I heard filled me with horror. A French doctor from a small resort on the coast of Corsica told us of the emergence of a germ which had become resistant to all commonly used antibiotics. It was spreading among bathers in the beautifully clear sea along the beaches of the island. The infections occurred immediately below some newly built holiday villa complexes that had not yet been connected to the sewage system, so they relied on septic tanks. As they all had washing machines and dish washers, the effluent was full of detergent which prevented normal decomposition of waste. The virulent organisms which seeped into the soil were then washed into the nearby sea by the rain.

Pseudomonas of various types has spread from the Mediterranean to the swimming pools of Europe and elsewhere, as well as other organisms such as *Staphylococcus aureus*, which produces distinctive golden pus.

We also see cases where the treatment with antibiotics has been very successful indeed, perhaps too successful, as it has killed off all the germs in the ear canal including the "good" ones that inhabit our bodies symbiotically. This leaves the ear devoid of germs, favourable or unfavourable, but open to settlement by other invaders. It is fungi such as the white *Candida albicans*, better known as thrush, and the painful, black *Aspergillus niger* which are difficult to eradicate since they are immune to antibiotics.

Infection of the outer ear is called *otitis externa* and its symptoms include deafness together with pain and discharge. These three symptoms may appear in varying proportions. Sometimes the infection is not acute and the pain more tolerable, maybe disappearing altogether. All is not well, however, as the disease is not cured but instead has entered an insidious and chronic phase. The skin becomes increasingly thickened and the canal narrows. Deafness is now the main symptom and is very difficult to treat. Even a hearing aid cannot always be fitted into a swollen, moist, canal and the plastic mould may well make the irritation worse.

Sometimes the infection is in the form of a boil which may be so painful that even chewing or opening the mouth can be unbearable.

3.1.3 *Foreign bodies*

Like the doctor in *Captain Correlli's Mandolin*, I have removed many foreign bodies from people's ears. Most of them have been from children but once I found a pearl in the ear of a woman in her 50s. She was amazed as she remembered her mother looking for it when the string of her necklace had broken, and yet the woman could not recall what she was doing when the necklace broke that would cause one of the pearls to lodge in her ear. The story had remained part of her family lore as it had taken place in the street and when passers-by had tried to help her mother, who was kneeling down scratching between the flagstones, she had replied, "It's all right I am only looking for pearls." One well-meaning person had called a policeman saying that there was a mad woman in charge of a little girl.

Why children put things in their ears is a matter for psychologists, but it is very common. Although stuffing from toys is easy to remove with tweezers, pearls or slippery pieces of plastic are impossible to grasp and can often be pushed in further, damaging the eardrum.

Adults often leave cotton wool buds which have broken off while they are trying to clean their ears and occasionally the tympanic membrane has been damaged as a result.

In the 1960s a girl once came to me, complaining that her hearing was muffled, but I could find nothing wrong on examination. Her eardrums actually looked better than normal as they glistened luminously, reflecting the light like a mirror. I suspected that there might be a psychological cause for her insistence that her hearing was inadequate.

Under the operating microscope's light beam her tympanic membrane gleamed even more brightly as it was magnified almost 20 times. I gently prodded the membrane and suddenly the whole surface cracked into opaque little segments like a car windscreen shattered by a pebble. She said at once that she could hear better than before.

It turns out that, in order to produce the *bouffant* or "bee-hive" effect that was fashionable in those days, it was necessary to backcomb the hair and glue it in place by means of a spray, some of which occasionally entered the ear canal. It formed a film over the tympanic membrane, thus interfering with its vibration. Since it was transparent we were not immediately aware of its existence. A few drops of spirit dissolved it away.

I saw this again in a very old character actress. She admitted to being well over 80 but she was always in demand for television. She had only a few wisps of hair left and the makeup people tried to make the most of it by spraying it with the same fixative as used in the *bouffant*. Everyone assumed that the resulting hearing loss was due to her age rather than an external factor.

Now that swimming is so popular I often find bits of ear plugs that have become detached in the ear canal.

3.1.4 *Misshapen canal*

As with every part of our anatomy, there is a wide variety in the shape of the ear canal.

Although a narrow passage will not, in itself interfere with the hearing, there is no doubt that it is more easily obstructed by wax, and that mild eczema or even dandruff can block it.

Occasionally we find little bony growths called osteoma. They are said to be particularly prevalent among swimmers. These are entirely benign, but however harmless, they can cause hearing loss when water or wax gets trapped behind them.

3.2 Disease of the Middle Ear

3.2.1 *Glue ear*

"He must be a late developer," my mother said one day, when I came home from school with a story about one of my classmates. "Like his older brother."

My news had been about a boy who had always sat at the back of the classroom and made no progress. Every now and again he would explode with boredom and do something outrageous. On the other hand he was very good-natured most of the time so the teacher tolerated his interruptions.

Year after year Victor had been placed at the bottom of the class results until one year, when we were aged about nine, and he came top in geography, an event so extraordinary that I reported it home.

Looking back now, I suspect that Victor simply could not hear very well in the classroom. A similar situation was apparent in Winston Churchill who once boasted that when he took the entrance examination for his preparatory school he had handed in a blank sheet of paper. In fact, his intelligence was apparent very early and the most likely explanation must be that he simply had not heard the question.

Indeed, I suspect that there were many children who suffered in this way because of a condition we now call *glue ear*. The condition was not recognised until the end of the 1950s because the hearing loss was never very severe, it fluctuated and was not present all the time. The condition tends to get better by the age of nine. Before the audiometer became available, precise records of hearing levels could not be kept, and without the operating microscope, an adequate view of the tympanic membrane was not possible.

As these children often performed badly in their early years at school, and then suddenly flourished, they were known as "late developers". On the other hand there can be little doubt that academic potential was lost forever by those who could not catch up and failed the 11-plus examination on which a person's future depended. This was more likely to happen among those who came from disadvantaged families.

If glue ear is present in the infant he may suffer a delay in developing speech, and in the past may well have been considered mentally subnormal. This actually led to a curious belief that removing the adenoids could sometimes "cure" retardation. Critics of the past suggest that it was venality among surgeons anxious to pocket fees. Old medical books, however, show how well meaning these people were and offer a clue to what happened then and a caution for us today.

Glue ear means that fluid, usually thick mucus, is trapped in the middle ear as a result of blocked Eustachian tubes which normally let air in from the space at the back of the nose. This space can be blocked by enlarged fleshy growths called adenoids which are present to some degree in all small children but only occasionally are swollen or inflamed enough to cause trouble.

The ear, filled with this glue-like mucus is not able to function very well and a child who cannot hear before he has developed speech will be considerably behind. Today we will label the child "speech-delayed" and not "language-delayed" as we have learnt to make the distinction between speech and language but it is not surprising that in the past they would simply say that the child was "retarded" which, in the literal sense of the word, I suppose he was.

A child with enlarged adenoids will keep his mouth open as he cannot breathe through the nose and is also likely to dribble. With the mucus, too, trickling down from the nostrils, his appearance is hardly prepossessing and this tends to upset the parents. In the past this would have confirmed the suggestion that he is retarded, especially if there is also delay in speaking.

Removing the adenoids and infected tonsils meant the tubes could drain, letting air pass into the middle ear and restore the hearing, allowing the child to breathe properly and eventually learn to speak. The child would have been cured of his "retardation".

Good doctors would, through experience, have been able to recognise the child who could be "cured" in that way and the one who could not, and would recommend surgery appropriately. Poor doctors may not have been able to tell the difference and, no doubt, there would also have been the venal surgeon who would, perhaps, have said, "I cannot promise, but I can try!" and operated on everyone he could get his hands on.

3.2.1.1 *Symptoms and signs of glue ear*

There are two symptoms of glue ear: deafness and earache.

Deafness is rarely severe and in the very young child it may be apparent only when speech delay becomes obvious. Between the ages of two and five it may not arouse suspicion at all and present simply as a recalcitrant child.

> "He only does what he's told if I shout at him!" or
> "He drives us mad turning the television up so loud!"

The school-age child may fail to progress and be inattentive or even disruptive. Teachers today are aware of this condition and screening tests are carried out at school.

The hearing fluctuates, however, so that a child who is sent for testing in the summer months may be normal and the school and parents wrongly reassured. I have known many children whose hearing was good during the holidays when they went to the clinic and who were deaf during the term so that they suffered years of educational failure before anyone realised.

Earache is not always present but when it is, it draws attention to the condition. The pain can be severe but it does not last very long as it is due to reduced pressure in the ear and is very similar to what happens in the airplane on landing.

The doctor may be able to see the fluid if the drum is thin, especially if it is yellowish in colour or if there is a fluid level. Sometimes the drum only appears dull, or it may look sucked in or "retracted".

Tuning fork tests show conductive deafness and audiometry will indicate the level of hearing loss, while tympanometry will produce the flat curve typical of glue ears.

3.2.1.2 *Treatment*

We may advise to do nothing, and some parents follow the advice. If the hearing loss is slight, it often reverts to normal, and if the child is given one-to-one attention so that speech is not delayed and there are minimal problems at school, it is quite possible to gently guide him or her through the years until the glue ear disappears. Some parents also try dietary changes, such as excluding dairy products.

On the other hand, if the child's speech is delayed, or if he is not doing well at school, and especially if he suffers from severe and frequent earache, it is not fair to withhold treatment.

Antibiotics, antihistamines and a group of drugs which loosen mucus called *mucolytic agents* have been tried and some children have improved. It remains uncertain, however, if it is the medication which has been effective or if they would have got better anyway.

It is also possible, under an anaesthetic, to make a tiny incision in the eardrum and suck out the mucus. This is called a *myringotomy* and at first we thought that was all that was necessary, but we soon found that the glue invariably returned.

It is not just a question of getting rid of the glue, because that was only the result of the middle ear being deprived of ventilation through Eustachian tube blockage. Other than *adenoidectomy*, removing the adenoids, not much can be done to unblock that tube so an alternative channel must be made to let air enter the cavity.

This is commonly done by inserting a little plastic tube called a *grommet* in an incision made in the drum to suck out the glue. The tubes have *flanges* so as to ensure the grommet does not fall in or out (Figure 12).

So long as the grommet is in place and air can enter the middle ear it is protected from mucus and the pain and deafness it may cause, but as the grommet is made of foreign material the body tends to reject it. The way it is rejected prevents it leaving a hole and, apart from a tiny scar, the drum returns to normal. Usually the grommet stays in place between six months and a year, but it sometimes survives much longer, in which case the patient is lucky as the biggest problem is early rejection which results in recurring glue and repeated surgery.

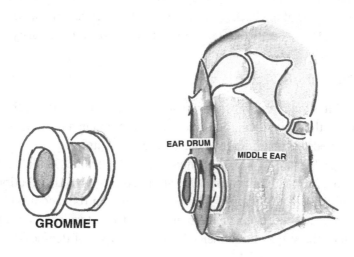

GROMMET

EAR DRUM

MIDDLE EAR

Figure 12. Grommet in tympanic membrane.

If this happens too frequently, it is possible to place a different type of tube with a bigger flange giving it a T-shape, but there is a greater likelihood of infection from swimming. Although it is commonly rejected in the same manner as a grommet, it may sometimes have to be removed, in which case the hole remains and the drum has to be closed by a graft. This rarely happens.

Myringotomy and grommet insertion is a very common and successful procedure which is mostly free from complication. Children are able to swim without ear plugs and infection usually troubles only a minority, and even then it is usually only a painless discharge which responds quickly to antibiotic ear drops. Removing adenoids at the same time is only necessary if they are enlarged.

3.2.1.3 *Glue ear in adults*

Glue ear occurs much less frequently in adults, and flying is a major cause, especially if the traveller has a cold.

The treatment is antibiotics taken together with decongestants, which can be in the form of pills or nose drops. In most people it clears within two weeks but occasionally it persists, and myringotomy with grommet insertion is required, just as in children.

We have to exclude malignancy when glue ear affects adults, as a tumour can grow at the back of the nose and that is what blocks the tubes. The doctor always keeps that possibility in mind despite its rarity.

3.2.2 *Otosclerosis*

2% of whites and Asians suffer from otosclerosis; it is rarer among Africans. In the United Kingdom we expect more than a million people to have inherited this condition and are deaf as a result.

After the Second World War, hearing aids became available in the United Kingdom and half those who attended the NHS distribution centres suffered from otosclerosis. When surgery was introduced this changed dramatically and the nature and management of otosclerosis led to the evolution of the surgical treatment of all other types of deafness.

In 1741 the Italian anatomist Antonio Valsalva was carrying out an autopsy on a deaf person so he was particularly interest in the ear. Most of its structure was already relatively well known and Valsalva was familiar with the eardrum and with the three tiny bones, the hammer, the anvil and the stirrup or stapes which conduct the sound vibrations across the middle ear.

He noticed, despite its minute size, that the little ossicle was solidly fixed and did not move however much he prodded it. Valsalva realised that this must have been the cause of the man's deafness as there was no way such a stapes could transmit sound vibrations. Later, doctors became aware that the fixation that interfered with the movement of the stapes was due to bone being laid down just where its footplate should be free and loose to vibrate back and forth in the oval window.

There was unease in the 1950s as genetics were coming to the fore and it was found that otosclerosis was not only inherited, but passed on as a dominant feature to most children of an affected person. This raised a question as most of those attending the new hearing aid centres were women.

Sex-linked transmission of congenital diseases was well known. In haemophilia, a condition understood at the time, the mother is the carrier but only the son is affected by the disease. A daughter might be a carrier but her second X chromosome would come from, presumably, an unaffected father. In the 1950s, it was not clear why women should be affected so much more frequently. During my student days it remained a mystery which deepened when a friend failed his surgical exams and could only find a job that took him to a small Arab sheikhdom.

He wrote to tell me that he had made a discovery: all those deafened by otosclerosis in the community were men; it seemed the local women having escaped it altogether. He was very excited as he expected that this extraordinary finding, the opposite of what occurred in the West, would lead to his past failures being forgiven. He investigated the phenomenon by seeking out the deaf men in their own homes. What he found, in his own words, was:

> "….their houses were full of deaf women! They were sitting around unable
> to hear a thing as they went around their daily activities: sewing, cooking

and doing the household chores. These women were the deaf men's sisters and when I counted them there were as many deaf women as there were men and they were more severely affected. When I asked why they had not been brought to see me I was told that women did not need to hear in order for them to get about their daily lives. Apparently they were better off that way."

Cultural and social factors had distorted our statistics as men and women were everywhere equally afflicted. The difference was that the deafness was less severe in men so, in Britain, they did not bothered to seek help at a time when none was really available. Pregnancy was what made the deafness so much worse in women so it became clear that we were dealing with a hormonal factor as well as a genetic one.

Although it occasionally appears unexpectedly, there is almost always a strong family history, as it can be inherited from either parent, and siblings are usually also affected.

Deafness often begins in the early 20s, or even the teens, and progresses so gradually that the person accommodates, subconsciously learning to lip-read, so that the hearing loss may not be seen to be a problem until the late 30s or 40s.

Since each subsequent pregnancy speeds up the progression of hearing loss, women tend to seek help sooner; this was especially true once hearing aids and later surgery became available.

Occasionally it affects only one ear but usually the other side loses the hearing in due course too. Tinnitus is often present and a few people also get vertigo.

It has been said that there are more cases of otosclerosis in areas of low fluoride in the water and this has led to treatment with fluoride tablets but I have not found the evidence convincing.

3.2.2.1 *Surgical treatment*

The story of the surgical treatment of this condition is also the story of modern otological surgery and the story of my working life. As soon as Valsalva had shown that deafness could be caused by fixation of the stapes, it was inevitable that surgeons would begin to poke about in patients' ears, attempting to prod it into movement with long needles.

The results must have been poor, not least because they could not see what they were doing. Many of the doctors could not distinguish properly between conductive and perceptive deafness, and most cases of conductive deafness, before antibiotics, were likely to be due to infection rather than otosclerosis so the chances are that they often selected the wrong patients.

Nevertheless there were some reports that hearing had been restored and hopes persisted for centuries, encouraged by the rare successful episodes.

It was only in the 19th century that a French surgeon, Camille Miot, presented an extraordinary collection of cases to the Royal Academy in Paris. What was striking was not just the large number of patients they had operated on, but the detailed description of exactly what they had done. They published drawings of the fine, needle-like instruments they had devised, with different curves and with tiny hooks, similar to those we use today.

They pushed their needles through the eardrum and prodded around what they thought was the stapes until it moved and the patient was able to hear. It is remarkable that they could do this at all without anaesthesia or magnification and electric lighting. Not surprisingly, however, the operation did not take on and the idea behind it lay dormant again for another century when a fortuitous event took place.

It was 1952 and magnification through the operating microscope was available; anaesthesia, both general and local, had arrived and antibiotics were there to ward off infection. Dr Sam Rosen of New York too was there and what happened, according to him was "chance favouring the prepared mind".

He told me all this at a medical meeting, after which I had missed the coach taking us to an evening event and I ended up, rather desolately, in an empty hotel dining room. Dr Rosen, then the most famous surgeon in the world, had also missed the coach and, inviting me to join him, talked to me for the rest of the evening.

When I got back to my room I wrote down as much as I could remember as I thought it may be of historical interest.

Dr Rosen said that he had devised an incision to enter the middle ear avoiding the tympanic membrane altogether by cutting the skin of the canal wall. I was already familiar with this as we called it "Rosen's Incision".

He told me that while he was operating inside the ear of a deaf patient for something unrelated to the hearing, his hand had slipped. His heart stopped, he said, when he felt a slight but quite definite crack and he withdrew his instrument instantly asking the patient, who was awake and had had a local anaesthetic, whether he was alright. The patient, amazed and delighted, announced that he could suddenly hear everything.

All the efforts since Valsalva had led to success, and this time the "stapes mobilisation" operation, though still carried out by prodding and scratching, spread like wildfire as the surgeon could now see what he was doing. Within a short time it led to further advances.

Rosen himself was still embattled when he told me his story. I was on the verge of my own career, and he was at the height of his, so I could hardly believe his tale of insecurity resulting, I imagined, from the poverty of his immigrant childhood in the tenements of Syracuse, in up-state New York, and later from the jealousy of many colleagues. There seems to have been a political side to it too. He had actively supported the left wing Henry Wallace for president against Harry S. Truman and sheltered the black singer Paul Robeson, a communist, in his own home at the height of McCarthyism. Unlike so many who lost their jobs, Rosen was one of the few who could cure deafness so his ostracism had been only social, but it still rankled.

Soon, a young surgeon from Memphis, Tennessee, called John Shea Jr went a step further in the story by removing the stapes all together. He covered the hole he had made in the solidified footplate with a piece of vein and attached a plastic piston to the incus, thus replacing the fixed ossicle with a mobile artificial one (Figure 13).

I met John Shea at breakfast at an Oxford college where we were both staying soon after I had just started training. I was awed by the presence of this great man having coffee though he was modest enough and seemed to be trying to encourage me. I suppose that is why he told me he had made a million dollars which seemed an incredible sum but I had nothing to say as we did not know how to discuss money in England then.

His operation was called *stapedectomy* and, despite many variants, has remained the standard surgical treatment for otosclerosis though over the years the hole in the stapes footplate is made as small as possible, so as to diminish leakage of inner ear fluid. With all the variants and improvements,

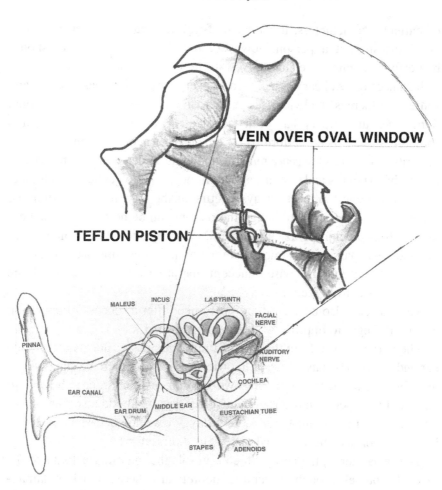

Figure 13. Stapedectomy. Shea Teflon piston replaces stapes.

we are still not far from the original breakthroughs of Sam Rosen and John Shea Jr. Stapes surgery forced surgeons to use the operating microscope and it helped to introduce "spare part surgery" to the 20th century.

3.2.2.2 *Risks and complications of stapedectomy*

As operations go, stapedectomy is relatively successful and free from risk. The worse thing that can happen is to lose the hearing altogether, which we call a "dead ear". Statistics show that dead ear occurs in less than 2%

of patients. Nonetheless, it cannot be forgotten that if it happens it is a 100% disaster to that person. However small the risk, no operation should be performed unless the alternatives are less acceptable.

Instances of dead ear are recorded in every surgeon's series of cases and sometimes there is an obvious cause, for example a post-operative infection. Sometimes the surgery has been technically exceptionally difficult, and sometimes it has been performed by an inexperienced surgeon, but in the majority of disasters the cause remains uncertain. A dead ear may be accompanied by dizziness and tinnitus, although these tend to get better with time.

Some dizziness almost always occurs in the first few days after the stapedectomy operation, although the patient can be helped with medication such as prochlorperazine (Stemetil). Driving should be avoided until dizziness has passed. It is impossible to say how long this takes as everyone is different, but it is wise to accept that at least two weeks should be set aside for convalescence.

Tinnitus can also become more prominent after a successful operation but it will begin to improve as hearing is regained.

The nerve of taste from the side of the tongue passes across the middle ear and it has to be pushed aside in order to have access to the stapes. This usually stretches it and sometimes we have to cut it in order to be able to carry out the operation properly. This often results in odd taste sensations but these tend to diminish after a few days or weeks; occasionally it can be a few months before normal taste sensation returns.

The facial nerve, the nerve which controls the muscular activity of the face, also passes through the ear and theoretically there is a risk of damaging it in any ear operation. This leaves an unaesthetic appearance but is very unlikely in stapedectomy.

Although the patient needs to be informed of the risks so that he or she can decide what to do, it is wrong to exaggerate them, as stapedectomy has been one of the most successful operations ever devised.

A curious point emerged later when magnetic resonance imaging (MRI) scans were introduced, as these cannot be done if there are any metal implants in the body. Other scans, for example a CT scan are available so it does not matter too much; nevertheless it is better to use plastic or ceramic devices rather than metal, which may be affected by the strong magnets of the MRI scanner.

3.2.2.3 *Management of otosclerosis*

Hearing aids only became widely available at around the same time as Rosen's mobilisation operation and as they were large, bulky boxes with wires and not very good amplifiers, surgery was definitely a more attractive proposition, despite the inevitable risks.

The situation is different now, as tiny aids can be hidden inside the ear canal. As a result, many patients prefer to try them before subjecting themselves to an operation, and some find them entirely satisfactory for a while. Nevertheless, as the hearing loss in otosclerosis is progressive, the moment ultimately comes when surgery is the only choice.

Whereas some people feel that one good ear is all they need, others feel that, although they can hear perfectly well in one ear, they need hearing in the other and request surgery. Everyone has different needs and even that may change with time and circumstance.

One woman, who was very deaf, had a successful result on one side and declined surgery on the other. Fifteen years later she wanted to hear with the other ear too, and when I asked why she had changed her mind after so many years, she explained that she had been elected mayor of her town.

"I have to chair meetings," she explained, "and I cannot hear what those sitting on the other side are saying."

It is best not to travel in aeroplanes immediately after surgery, even though in normal circumstances aircraft are well pressurised. I have had a number of patients over the years that flew back to their own country as soon as they left the hospital, and I supposed they must have been told not to pay any attention to my advice. As far as I am aware, nothing terrible happened to any of them, and it is possible that we can get over cautious.

Swimming can start again as soon as the eardrum has healed but I would exclude scuba diving to any depth forever.

3.2.3 *Otitis media: infection of the middle ear*

3.2.3.1 *Acute otitis media*

In the days before antibiotics, acute otitis media was a common and serious condition. Children in particular were often left deaf and sometimes died.

Infection can easily reach the ear from the nose following a cold or tonsillitis. The middle ear cavity fills with pus under pressure and the drum bursts to let it out. Infection may spread to the bone behind the ear, the mastoid bone, to cause *mastoiditis*. In the past, if the abscess which had formed was not quickly drained, it would turn into meningitis or spread to the brain and would invariably be fatal.

The mastoid abscess is drained through a cut made behind the ear known as Wilde's Incision after the Dublin surgeon who had introduced it, Sir William Wilde. Incidentally, it is ironic that his own son, the playwright Oscar Wilde, died from just such an infection, while spending his last days in a dingy hotel in Paris. Dismal or not the Hotel d'Alsace in Saint-Germain des Prés was expensive for the writer who is reputed to have said "I am dying beyond my means" before he passed away in room number 16. Today it is a four star establishment called "l'Hotel" and it proudly broadcasts its connection with Oscar Wilde.

When I was growing up in Cairo, I played with many of the children in our building, the Baehler building, and it was common for upper respiratory infection to spread from one child to another, often leading to earache. One year, two little English boys became seriously ill and there was silence in the block when the specialist came to their apartment. The word had got round that he was operating there and then as it was too late to get the boys to the hospital, and all the doors stood open to learn what was happening.

Unfortunately, they both died, just as my younger brother was being taken to the hospital for surgery for the same thing. Draining the mastoid had not been enough and the specialist explained to my parents that there was only one hope other than a miracle.

There was a new medicine that was said to be miraculous. A military doctor from the Scottish Hospital had told our specialist that when Churchill had contracted pneumonia during his visit to the Eighth Army, he had been cured within hours. The drug had been used during the landings in Sicily and there was some in Egypt but it was entirely in the hands of the military and he had no means of getting any.

The hours that followed have lengthened in my memory, as time can appear elastic: it seemed as though days and weeks went by, rather than hours. My parents went to beg in different quarters, approaching government officials, Army personnel and anyone they knew who had some sort of contact or connection. My father offered money, which was all he had to offer, only to be told that the wonder drug could not be bought.

Somehow they obtained a vial containing what was now their only hope as my brother was getting worse. My mother had been told that it had to be administered every three hours intramuscularly, and the doctor had shown her how to give the injections. She spent the night with the alarm clock by her side, but I know she did not sleep.

By the morning the temperature had gone down and the following day my brother was better, though no one was sure how long the course of medication should be. It was thought that three days might be enough.

The new medicine, I was told, was called *penicillin*. After that nothing was ever the same in the medical world, and everything seemed possible, as antibiotics not only cured people, but allowed us to invade the body to repair damage and introduce spare parts without causing infection.

In my whole career as an ENT surgeon I have never seen a single death resulting from an acute ear infection. It is a thing of the past. The deafness in acute middle ear infection seems hardly important, as the symptoms are dominated by severe earache and a raised temperature. Often the infecting organism is a virus allied to that which produces colds and the illness resolves without perforation or other more serious damage over the next couple of days.

If the symptoms persist for longer than that, it is wiser to start antibiotics while watching for possible complications. Perhaps my personal memories loom too large, as some medical specialists condemn the widespread use of antibiotics.

Earache is usually the result of pressure changes whether there is an infection or not. Anyone who has been in an aeroplane with a number of small children will have noticed how they all start crying as the plane descends. Sitting them up and giving them something they can suck as well as nose drops helps.

3.2.3.2 *Chronic otitis media*

There are two types of chronic infection that have traditionally been known as "safe" and "unsafe", although of course no disease can be considered completely safe.

Bad acute infections often happen when the tympanic membrane has perforated and failed to heal. From time to time the middle ear cavity, now open to the elements, particularly to water, will become re-infected and drain pus so we call it "chronic *suppurative* otitis media" or, in doctors' shorthand, CSOM. Very often these repeated bouts of infection result in damage to the tiny ossicles that transmit sound vibrations. They literally rot away and the most vulnerable is the long arm of the incus which loses contact with the stapes so that the vibrations cannot be passed on and hearing is lost. Although chronically infected ears do not necessarily hurt, quite frequently the infection becomes more acute in which case it may become painful.

When the ear is discharging, treatment is with antibiotics taken by mouth or in the form of drops directly into the ear or both together. This usually restores the ear to its quiescent state. On the other hand the tympanic membrane remains perforated and therefore open to repeated infection; often the hearing continues to deteriorate as a result of further damage and scarring of the ossicular chain.

The alternative is surgery, as the perforation can be repaired by a graft and the ossicular chain reconstructed, but as the ear is "safe" it remains a matter of choice. Some people decide to leave things as they are and avoid activities that will exacerbate an infection, such as swimming, and treat recurrent infections when they come.

3.2.3.3 Cholesteatoma

Unsafe chronic otitis media is a sinister and dangerous disease as it leads to gradual destruction of the hearing and, if left unchecked, can cause facial paralysis and even death from meningitis or brain abscess.

The name given to the condition, cholesteatoma, is wrong and misleading; nevertheless it has stuck over the years, despite attempts to give it a more appropriate one.

The misunderstanding started with early autopsies of people who had died following ear infections, as many were found to have a white, soft, round ball, like a pearl, in the middle ear cavity which appeared to have eroded and destroyed the adjoining structures. Parts of the ossicular chain had often disappeared and sometimes even the facial nerve would be damaged so, not surprisingly, they thought it was a tumour eating them away and, as they classified growths according to the tissue they had arisen from by adding the suffix -*oma*, they did so here.

The exact tissue to which this particular tumour had grown from was not known, and caused great puzzlement. When the growth was inspected with a microscope, only what looked like cholesterol crystals could be seen. They did not know what to make of this "tumour" and so they called it a "cholesterol tumour" or *cholesteatoma*, and the name has remained, although we now know that it is no tumour at all but simply a bag of skin. The layers of skin naturally peel off inside this bag, and simply rot into a mass of soft white dead tissue which disintegrates into a fatty mess where cholesterol crystals form, giving the distinctive microscopic appearance which led to the name.

What causes this to happen is still uncertain, although in a few cases it may be a small quantity of skin trapped in the ear region of the embryo. However, in most cases it seems to be a pocket that creeps in from outside, getting bigger and bigger; we therefore call it a "retraction pocket". This begins in the upper part of the middle ear and the opening of the retraction pocket is usually clearly seen at the top of the drum. We call it the *attic region* and a perforation in that position (Figure 14) is the clue to its sinister or "unsafe" nature as the "safe" perforations lie in the centre of the drum.

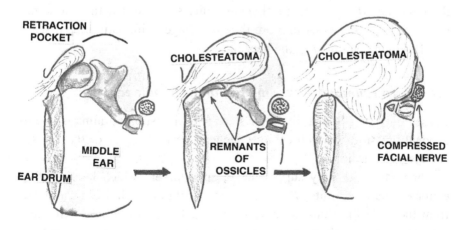

Figure 14. Cholesteatoma.

The rotting mass of dead skin gets infected with an evil-smelling discharge and deafness follows due to the destruction of the ossicles. When it becomes painful it is an ominous sign of impending catastrophe, inviting early surgery.

Facial paralysis sometimes appears. Although there are many other causes of facial palsy, when it is associated with deafness or discharge it suggests a call to the surgeon.

The same applies to vertigo. Although this may be caused by many things, if pain or discharge is present, cholesteatoma should be suspected. That unpleasant disease can also erode into the inner ear, and not only destroy the hearing but also balance.

As soon as these facts were understood the *radical mastoidectomy operation* was devised. I was initially taught to do it with a hammer and chisel but we do it now with a high speed electric drill and it involves removing the tympanic membrane and what is left of the ossicular chain, creating a cavity which includes the middle ear and the mastoid bone. As there is no eardrum, it is open to the outside so that when we look into the ear canal we see right into the empty cavity and are able to clean it out and inspect it regularly. The French aptly call the operation *evidement*, or "emptying".

Radical mastoidectomy does not spare the hearing, but as cholesteatoma is life-threatening, there is no option but surgery. Over the years, however, techniques have evolved which have allowed us to reconstruct the ossicular transmission mechanism quite successfully, though sometimes we have to do this in more than one stage, eliminating the disease first and then dealing with the hearing.

3.2.4 *Barotrauma: pressure injuries to the middle ear*

Caused by flying, scuba diving or slaps and kisses, barotrauma is due to unequal pressure between cavities such as the middle ear or the sinuses and the outside air.

Our bodies can only survive in an environment which keeps within extremely narrow limits. We cannot be too cold or too hot or we die, but from the time that humans covered themselves with animal skins and built their own shelters we have learnt to extend the range of outside temperature in which we can survive. The air we breathe has to contain a minimum amount of oxygen but technological advances have allowed us to take it with us under the sea or in outer space.

The same narrow limits apply to pressure.

The atmosphere consists of molecules of air which are kept close to the earth by gravity. If this were absent, the air would be allowed to float away into space. The strength of gravity is greatest the closer we are to the centre of the earth and so the air is denser near the surface than it is at 30,000 feet on the top of Mount Everest, for instance, or when we are flying at that height.

The pressure at sea level is that exerted by a column of 50 miles of air bearing on top of us. We can call it 1 atmosphere. Different specialists, such as weathermen and divers, prefer other units for technical reasons. Thus, 1 atmosphere is the same as 14.7 pounds per square inch (psi) or 101.3 kilopascal (kPa).

As the air is so much less dense at the top of Mount Everest the pressure there is only 0.25 (a quarter of 1 atmosphere) or 4.12 psi.

On the other hand, if we dive under the sea, the pressure is not only that of the 50-mile column of air but also that of the column of sea water beneath it. At a depth of 30 feet the pressure is therefore twice that at sea level, or 2 atmospheres, so we refer to it as *ambient pressure* rather than atmospheric pressure.

3.2.4.1 *Flying*

The outside pressure on an airplane changes from the 14.7 psi at sea level, to only 1.5 psi when it is cruising. The air is too "thin" at that level to sustain human life, not to speak of the temperature, and this relative vacuum would suck out all human tissues to the point where body cavities would burst. This means that the pressure in the cabin must be artificially maintained and the air in it must contain enough oxygen for adequate respiration. This is done by taking in outside air, compressing it and regulating it by vents which let the air out at an appropriate rate.

Regulations require that all commercial aircraft maintain a cabin pressure of a minimum of 10.9 psi, which is equivalent to an altitude of about

8,000 feet. Cruising cabin pressure tends to be at between 6,000 and 8,000 feet, equivalent to Denver, Colorado (more than 5,000 feet) and Machu Picchu in Peru (almost 8,000 feet).

This means that when the aircraft lands, the pressure change from cruising altitude to surface pressure is still considerable and the *rate of change* between them is very important. If it is too rapid there would be problems with the ears, sinuses and respiratory system. The rate of change should be equivalent to not more than 5 metres per second (1,000 feet per minute) during ascent and 2.3 metres per second (450 feet per minute) on descent.

The middle ear is a cavity, and if the pressure inside is not equal to that outside, it would be damaged as the tympanic membrane would be sucked in or blown out depending on the direction of the pressure difference.

The middle ear avoids damage to some extent, as it communicates with the outside at the back of the nose through the Eustachian tube and air may come in and out as necessary. However it cannot do so freely, as the tube acts as a valve which lets the air out relatively easily but not back in.

This means that there is usually not much of a problem when the aeroplane takes off. The air pressure in the cabin diminishes as we rise but the difference with that in the middle ear quickly equalises as air escapes through the Eustachian tube.

This is not the case on descent, particularly if the rate at which the pressure changes is too rapid, as the air cannot re-enter the middle ear through the valve-like tube. We have to take active measures to open it, for example swallowing or yawning. When we swallow or yawn we contract the muscles of the palate attached to the soft walls of the tube, tugging at them and pulling them open. If we pinch the nostrils closed while we are doing that, the pressure at the back of the nose will increase, encouraging the air into the middle ear. That is called the Valsalva manoeuvre after the same man who noted that the stapes was fixed in some deaf patients.

If the tissues are inflamed and swollen, for instance when we fly with a cold, the situation on landing is made much worse as the passage is narrowed, as well as blocked with mucus, and the air may not get back in at all.

When that happens, the pressure is so low compared to the outside that the eardrum will get painfully sucked in, and the hearing badly muffled. Occasionally the thin tympanic membrane may even burst, or blood and fluid may be drawn into the middle ear from the surrounding tissues so it is wise to try to prevent this happening by using a decongestant spray about 20 minutes before landing to reduce the swelling, and then carrying out the Valsalva manoeuvre every few minutes as the aircraft loses height.

3.2.4.2 Scuba diving

People have been free-diving for food, pearls, coral and sponges as far back as human memory. Free-diving is done by holding the breath for as long as possible, but this is rarely for more than a minute or so due to lack of oxygen.

Herodotus tells the story of a Greek man named Scyllis who caused great damage to the Persian fleet by pretending to be drowned, and prowling about under water, interfering with Xerxes' ships. He was able to do this by breathing through a hollow read while keeping his head below the surface, in an early form of what we would now call snorkelling. We can keep this up a long time but we cannot go very deep.

Diving bells were first used in the 16th century, later along with leather diving suits with air pumped into them. As they went deeper, the pressure increased, requiring strong metal helmets and problems such as difficulty in deflating the lungs became more obvious. Meanwhile submarines were developed in the early 1860s with their own atmosphere maintained for temperature, pressure and oxygen; much as an aircraft cabin does but in reverse.

Individual divers have been able to carry their own supply of compressed air in canisters strapped to their backs from the middle of the 20th century. In the last few decades this has become an extraordinarily popular leisure activity. It has been estimated that there are some ten million divers worldwide who use self-carried underwater breathing apparatus (scuba); in the United States alone it is said that almost half a million licences are granted every year for recreational scuba diving.

Naturally, there are a number of health problems associated with scuba diving, but if training and proper standards are followed, scuba diving is a relatively safe sport. Sadly, it is not indicated for people who have trouble with their ears although nasal blockage can often be surgically corrected allowing the enjoyment of diving.

The problems with ears and scuba diving are similar to those experienced in flying: if the Eustachian tubes are blocked by a cold or from allergy the air cannot pass into the middle ear on descent and the tympanic membrane is sucked in. Divers call this "middle ear squeeze" and often the sinuses suffer as well. Symptoms tend to occur at a depth of only a few feet and if the pressure cannot be equalised easily by the Valsalva manoeuvre it is best to abandon the dive, as persistence may lead to rupture of the drum and vertigo which is even more dangerous. Inequality between middle and inner ear pressure will cause disorientation and may burst the thin membrane over the round window with the possibility of losing the hearing altogether.

Fewer ear problems are likely to occur during ascent but pressure on the drum has been known to cause "outward" rupture and vertigo has also happened.

Decompression sickness, also known as "the bends", is the result of dissolved gases coming out of solution and forming bubbles which can migrate all over the body and even cause death. This is something entirely different and unrelated to ear problems.

3.2.4.3 *Slaps and kisses*

A box on the ears with a clenched fist may be very painful and cause bleeding and even damage the pinna to give a "cauliflower ear" but it is unlikely to result in serious damage to the hearing.

A slap, however, may cause a pressure change in the ear canal and effects similar to other forms of barotrauma. I have seen a number of perforated eardrums in older people who claimed that it was the result of a slap administered by a teacher. This never occurs in schools in the United Kingdom now and most injuries to the tympanic membrane and middle ear due to blows and slaps are the result of what the police euphemistically call "a domestic".

Strangely, a more affectionate form of "domestic" which can also cause perforations is a kiss placed directly on the ear-hole!

Similar damage occurs in swimming pools, particularly among water-polo players as the impact of wet skin seals the ear-hole and brings about a pressure change.

The treatment is antibiotics and avoidance of getting water in the affected ear. In most cases the perforation heals spontaneously over six weeks to three months. If after that time there is no closure it is best to consider repair by means of a graft.

3.2.5 *Fractures*

Unfortunately the increase in road traffic accidents has made fractures of the temporal bone, which contains the ear, quite common.

Serious injuries may break into the inner ear in which case the deafness is complete and total and the hearing can never be recovered. Usually this is accompanied by dizziness which tends to recover, and often by tinnitus which behaves in its own unpredictable way. These fractures are always on one side only as a crack that goes right through the skull to the other side is unlikely to allow the victim to survive. Concussion without actual fracture through the inner ear may cause perceptive deafness, which may even recover to some extent if it is not total.

Some cases, however, result only in conductive deafness due to fracture or displacement of the little bones of the ossicular chain. That is why it is important to check the nature of the deafness after an accident in case it could be repaired by surgery.

There is also a rare a condition known as "brittle bone disease" or by its Latin name *fragilitas ossium* which is inherited as a dominant gene by both males and females. Bones fail to develop normal strength and elasticity and there are frequent fractures, even in the little bones of the middle ear, causing hearing loss. The deafness is made worse by a callus forming around the fracture site, often involving the footplate of the stapes. It becomes fixed, just like in otosclerosis (although it is a different condition), and a stapedectomy can restore the hearing. The ossicles, however, are so fragile that further fractures, of the incus for instance, may also interfere with the hearing.

3.2.6 *Middle ear reconstruction*

Reconstructing the mechanism of the middle ear to restore the hearing in conductive deafness has been the most successful and rewarding aspect of ear, nose and throat surgery in the second half of the 20th century.

The success was dependent on the development of the operating microscope which allows us to view the ossicular chain at a magnification of four, ten, sixteen or more times and it has also benefited from the availability of new materials which can replace the damaged ossicles.

3.2.6.1 *Tissue grafts*

Grafts can come from the patient himself, in which case they are called *autografts*. These grafts are not rejected, as the body does not see them as something foreign, so they can take very well provided they have an adequate blood supply. If they do not they will simply shrivel and reabsorb. Thin, superficial layers of skin can take if placed on a raw area even if they do not have a specific blood supply at all as they are fed directly from the bed on which they are placed. Thicker skin needs its own blood vessels and has to remain attached so we often refer to such arrangements as "flaps".

Bone is often used in the ear where the ossicles themselves can be repositioned in a different place, or a small piece of bone from elsewhere can replace a diseased structure. It is different from skin, however, as it consists not only of living cells, but of a calcium-based mineral which is what gives it strength and solidity. When we place a little bony autograft in the ear we expect that the cells of the surrounding tissues will grow into the mineral structure to give it life.

A graft taken from another person is called *a homograft*, and will be rejected as though it were a mouldering piece of wood unless powerful anti-rejection drugs are used. It is worth doing this if the graft is the kidney or the heart and lungs but not reasonable for transplanting an ear. On the other hand, tiny homografts such as ossicles, have worked very well without special medication. Grafts can also be taken from animal parts such as bovine amniotic membrane. They are called *xenografts* and, although they have been used in the ear, they have never been very popular as they did not give good results.

3.2.6.2 *Other materials*

Although attempts at giving some hearing after mastoid and cholesteatoma surgery have been made almost since that type of surgery began, it was only when stapedectomy for otosclerosis was introduced that a search for materials that would not get rejected began.

John Shea's first piston was a polyethylene tube simply because such tubing was easily available. The aim, however, was to find a material so inert that it would not be rejected, and a Teflon piston came into fashion. This has remained standard and I have used it myself ever since, but other pistons, such as stainless steel which work perfectly well, have been introduced; in many ways it is a matter of personal taste and preference of the surgeon.

There is a good reason to be glad for choosing to use a plastic device rather than a metal one. Since MRI scans have become a common procedure, I have had innumerable telephone calls from radiology departments who want to know what I had used in a particular patient 20 or 30 years ago. MRI scans are now so widely used that it is difficult to avoid them, but the radiologists do not like to place patients in their big magnets if they have a piece of steel implanted somewhere in their head.

The success of prostheses fixed onto the incus in stapedectomy was so great that we tried to attach plastic or metal pistons to the malleus too, in patients where the incus was missing. This did not work because when foreign material touched the drum or tissue other than the bone itself they were rejected. The immediate result may have been good but I remember too well my embarrassment when the patients returned with a piston that had literally fallen out of their ear.

For this implant, the profession turned to slivers of bone taken from the patient, but the search for a material that would not be rejected continued and an extraordinary array of materials was tried, including coral, whose consistency resembled bone in many ways. A new material made from calcium called apatite was introduced in an attempt to imitate the mineral part of bone. This has worked well and is still in use, but it "bonds" only with bone and is still rejected when it comes into contact with soft tissue such as the tympanic membrane. Nevertheless, a new word had entered our conversations somewhat surreptitiously and "bonding" came to mean a material that actually "stuck to things" rather than one that was simply not rejected.

Initially, as in the case of a wooden leg or of false teeth missing, inadequate parts could not be implanted at all but only applied to the surface of the body. When the way we react to foreign materials was understood, the search began for what might irritate the tissues so little that it would not be rejected if implanted, a substance so "inert" that the body would simply not notice it was there. That enterprise was successful, and plastics and stainless steel were used extensively, as well as porous materials like titanium, which is so inert that the cells of the surrounding tissues grow into its spaces binding it in place. Now we were on the brink of something else, and instead of something inert, it became necessary to look for a "bioactive" substance, which actively engaged in the metabolism of the body, "bonding" with it as muscle does to bone.

Then Larry Hench, a professor of material science at the University of Florida, introduced me to a novel concept and a new way of looking at the problem. Hench had discoverd a new material, a glass which he had named *Bioglass*®. He offered me the opportunity to collaborate in a project that culminated in the making of cone-shaped ossicular replacements which could easily be pared to the right size and shaped with a fine drill. These were given the name of *Douek–MED* (middle ear device) (Figure 15).

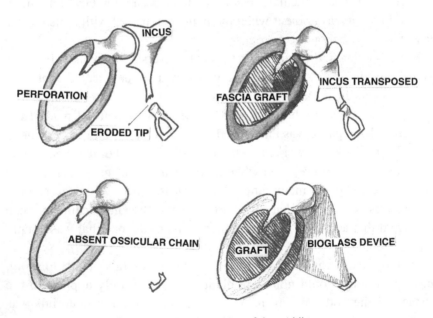

Figure 15. Reconstruction of the middle ear.

3.2.6.3 *Myringoplasty*

This is the name we give to the operation designed to close a perforation of the tympanic membrane by a graft.

Skin seemed, at first, to be the right material as the most superficial layer of the eardrum is itself skin, but the results were poor and the technique was quickly abandoned.

Segments of vein, the fascia that lies over muscle as well as the tissues that cover bone and cartilage, taken from the patient himself have all been successful and we can expect most of them to take.

3.2.6.4 *Ossiculoplasty*

The most common problem following infection is the destruction of the tip of the incus leaving a gap between the remains of the chain and the stapes so that sound vibrations are not transmitted. The rest of the incus can be removed and reshaped with a drill so that it can be replaced in a manner that will bridge the gap. If the incus has disappeared altogether then a replacement has to be found and that is where apatite or Bioglass® can be used. The latter is particularly helpful if the drum is missing too and has to be replaced by a graft. Absence of most of the stapes can happen, leaving only the footplate.

3.2.6.5 *Tympanoplasty*

This usually simply means that most of the middle ear or *tympanum* has to be replaced and represents a combination of myringoplasty with ossiculoplasty.

3.2.6.6 *Combined approach tympanoplasty*

When we feel confident that we have removed a cholesteatoma so completely that it will not recur, we can go on to graft a new drum and to reconstruct the hearing mechanism using shaped fragments of bone, or alternative materials to replace the ossicles (see Figure 15). This is called a *combined approach tympanoplasty*. Often we are not certain and we perform the operation in two stages, the first to excise the disease and close the drum with a graft, and the second, usually six months later, to check that it is free of cholesteatoma so that we may proceed with the reconstruction.

3.2.6.7 *Risks in ear surgery*

The aim in ear surgery is to end up with a safe, hearing ear. However, the surgery may fail due to the extent of the disease and the conditions we may find. The remains of the ossicular chain may be so bound up in scar tissue which may even have become ossified so that no surgery will be able to get everything moving. The blood supply of the region may be so poor that no graft will take and the tympanic membrane will remain perforated.

We can also make things worse and the ear may even end up totally deaf.

The facial nerve can be damaged as it passes through the middle ear, and although it can occur even in the best of hands when disease is very extensive, it happens only rarely. The most common cause, however, other than when tumours are involved, is lack of experience on the part of the surgeon.

Chapter 4

Perceptive or Neurosensory Deafness

Perceptive deafness results from impairment of the cochlea, or of the nerve of hearing, and also from malfunction in areas in the brain concerned with hearing. As the balance organ or labyrinth and its nerve are so closely related to the cochlea and the auditory nerve, disturbance of balance and hearing loss often occur together.

I attend committee meetings from time to time and on one of these occasions I was more interested than usual, as it was about nomenclature rather than money. The task was to change the name of *perceptive deafness* to something more suitable.

It took all day. Making a distinction between *perceptive* and *conductive* deafness had only become important when doctors were able to treat conductive deafness and now, again, modern technology had shown that perceptive deafness too should be subdivided. This type of deafness may be due to failure of the inner ear or cochlea, or of the nerve of hearing, and we realised that soon it may well be possible to treat the one and not the other, hence the need to separate the two. After all, the most valuable contribution that classification can make is to let us know whether anything can be done.

The discussion seemed interminable and I became conscious of the human need to change things or maybe just to change the names of things so as to give ourselves the illusion that we are moving ahead. Those in favour of change were adamant that we could not possibly retain *perceptive*, as it reeked of the past and we were all fearful of appearing out of date. Some suggested *neurosensory* instead while others thought that as the sense organ or cochlea came before the nerve, we should call it *senso-rineural*. Somebody else insisted it did not look right spelt that way.

I never found out the ultimate decision, or maybe I just forgot, for a particular usage is never entirely stable and during my career I have referred to both terms as the mood has taken me. I have not discarded the term *perceptive deafness* either, as, although "*neurosensory*" is useful when referring to the cochlea and the nerve, there is still an area which remains mysterious: sometimes when we fail to perceive sounds or understand their meaning it is the brain that is affected. No doubt this will be better understood now that we have functional magnetic resonance and positron emission scans which allow us to study the brain's activity in real time. The term *perceptive deafness* may find a role again.

4.1 Disease of the Inner Ear

The hearing organ or cochlea which forms part of the inner ear fails as we age and can be damaged by excessive noise. Some drugs too can cause harm while infection can destroy it altogether.

That the blood supply to the inner ear may be interrupted or haemorrhages occur into it is likely but usually unverified.

Ménière's disease is a condition which affects the whole inner ear and because it also affects balance, it poses special problems (see Section 4.1.8).

4.1.1 Presbyacusis or the effects of ageing

As we grow older we all gradually lose some hearing as part of the wear and tear of life, but the rate at which this happens varies from person to person. Although we do not know exactly what lies behind such differences, some of the differences are obvious.

We are not surprised, for instance, to find that those who have worked for years in noisy factories tend to deteriorate more rapidly than people who have lived quieter lives. When, in the 1960s, it was reported that the hearing of African Bushmen lasted longer than that of city dwellers it gave rise to much excited speculation. Was it the noise of civilisation which was responsible or was it that the Bushmen did not eat so many sweets? Or was it, perhaps, animal fat? All these are possible but there is one factor that tends to be brushed aside because it is difficult to face. We simply take after our parents, and whatever contribution anything else may make we can rarely escape our inherited destiny completely.

There is no medicine, either, that postpones the onset of ageing, but that does not mean we need not try to delay it by taking vitamins, trace elements or gingko biloba, even though there is no indisputable evidence that they make much difference. Treatment of other old age diseases, such as high blood pressure and raise cholesterol has been very successful in the sense that the complications of these conditions have been reduced, but no one has shown that hearing loss in particular can be postponed. Although *presbyacusis* or hearing loss from ageing is not a disease, it is disabling, and its effect on our lives needs to be minimised as we are not yet able to replace the failing organ. There is some indication that this may be possible one day but it will certainly not happen for a while. As life expectancy is greater each year, more of us will live longer than our parents and grandparents. This is all to the good, but it also means that we are likely to experience increasing hearing loss as the decades go by.

We lose the higher frequencies first, so that speech sounds such as "sss" and "fff" and the distinction between many consonants becomes inaudible, while the sounds that make up the vowels and contain lower frequencies can be heard perfectly well. In time the middle range of frequencies cannot be heard at conversational level either and eventually even the vowels become a problem. Such a pattern of hearing loss is by far the most common one but not the only one.

Losing the high frequencies means that although we may be able to hear, we do not do so clearly. When the number of nerve fibres and hearing cells has diminished, we may not be able to distinguish properly between one sound and another, adding to the lack of clarity. Amplification by a hearing aid does not always make speech clearer even though we may need it to hear anything at all.

Listening attentively and watching the lips carefully are still very important, even with the help of hearing aids. As the sound and vocabulary of spoken language alters with changing fashions, we become burdened with an extra difficulty in understanding as we get older — the typical evolution of language does not help us understand what coming generations are saying. This can be obvious when watching old films as the speech of our own childhood appears quite bizarre in today's ears. Other than these factors, the management of deafness in the elderly is not much different from that of other. Of course, there is the added difficulty of failing eyesight as so much depends on attention and lip-reading.

4.1.2 *Hazardous noise*

Loud sounds damage the inner ear and may cause tinnitus as well as hearing loss.

This happens as a result of exposure to the noise of machinery in the work place as well as the use of fire arms in the police, armed forces or as a sport. Excessively loud music has also caused much damage in recent years.

In the 1980s I travelled once a month to Brussels, joining colleagues from other countries as I represented the United Kingdom in what was then called the European Community. Our job was to decide what noise levels should be permitted in industry and on what basis compensation should be paid, though an official of the European Commission made clear to us right away that we could only recommend.

"After all," he had said at our first meeting, "you may say that no noise at all is the best environment for the workers' ears but without machinery we cannot make cars or drill holes."

We had to end up with reasonable recommendations taking into account the needs of industry as well as those of safety, and the difference could be made be up, as it were, by monetary compensation.

Our suggestions would then be passed on to another committee to see how it might be applied to factories without preventing them from functioning and then it would go to a third committee to put it into law. If what we recommended meant replacing old, unsafe factories by modern, quieter, and probably more productive ones or even closing them altogether, job losses may result. Although the community might recognise the benefits of our recommendations, it may wish to wait for a period of full employment before putting such excellent but costly measures into practice.

It was the first time that I had seen economic life expressed that way, but excessive noise has been with us ever since men struck flint stones to fashion implements in the Stone Age. That paradox was noted in Ecclesiastics:

> "without the smith, and the sound of constant hammering in his ears, a city cannot be inhabited." (Ecclesiastics 6:12)

Similar comments are common in antiquity, as in Martial's epigram from the first century which protests at the hammering that goes on "the whole day long".[2] Presumably, too, people have always protected their ears as best they could, though the first record that we have advising workers to do this in the book *De Morbis Artificum Diatriba.* This remarkable work, which translates as *Discourse on the Diseases of Workers,* dates from the very beginning of the 18th century and the age of enlightenment. It was written by Bernardino Ramazzini who taught medicine at Modena, and then at Padua, in Italy; we could consider him to be the founder of industrial medicine. He made other contributions to early epidemiology as he studied the spread of chickpea poisoning and malaria. Indeed he also strongly supported the use of cinchona bark which contains quinine to treat malaria rather than purgatives which had been the chief medicine since Galen. In his book, Ramazzini said that those who hammered copper for a living ultimately went deaf, and suggested that they protect themselves.

Even though the effects of noise have been known for so long, financial redress for damaged hearing belongs mainly to our own time and has come from the military, as well as industry. Compensation for injury as such (not specifically for hearing loss) has been mandatory since biblical times as the Law of Moses has been accepted as the moral basis of Western culture for many centuries. As interpreted in the Babylonian Talmud, if a master strikes a slave on the ear so that he is rendered deaf then he must give the slave his freedom, which was an expensive level of compensation at the time. This followed the general principles of punishment for physical injury from assault, but if someone screams in a person's ear, he is immune from punishment. Presumably this is because a scream is rarely loud enough to inflict a physical injury such as deafness and is more often considered a psychological insult.

---

[2] Martial *Epigrams*: Book XII.

Gunpowder explosions were known to deafen bystanders since they began being used in the 14th century. In the 18th century, Admiral Lord Rodney, who fought the French and the Spanish, was said to have been deafened when his ship, the *Formidable*, fired a broadside. Nevertheless, it was not until after the Second World War that the idea of compensation was considered.

One day, with thoughts of A.J. Cronin's *The Citadel* in mind, I went to visit one of the last old-fashioned iron foundries before it closed permanently. When I reached the railway station in Sheffield in the north of England and began to walk towards the foundry, I was conscious of a tremor under my feet; a repetitive vibration which transformed itself into a thudding sound as I got nearer.

Inside the black, fortress-like building I saw a vision akin to hell: enormous ladles poured out the liquid metal which radiated an intense heat. The worst of it all, however, was a huge hammer which was raised to the distant ceiling and then dropped down to forge the red-hot steel only to rise again, repeating the process endlessly, making me feel slightly dizzy as the pressure from the noise jarred my ears.

I was struck that conversations carried on regardless of the deafening sound, and it was clear that the workers could all lip-read at a considerable distance. Everyone there — from the owner, who had greeted me when I arrived, to the manager and the workers — was deaf. The foreman, who showed me round, told me that he had fought in the Battle of el-Alamein in the Second World War and recalled the continuous sound of explosions, adding that his father had served in the artillery in the First World War.

"Everyone was deaf in my family," he said. "Me granddad was deaf, me dad was deaf, me nan and me mam are deaf from working in the mills, where the spinning and weaving machines went *clickety-clack* all day. When I was a kid, all the women were gossiping away, non-stop, entirely by lip-reading."

"Well, at least it's over," I said. "The spell has been broken; it will all be robots now."

"I don't know," he replied. "My son plays drums in a rock band and you should hear their new loudspeakers."

Noise-induced deafness occurs in every walk of life. Obviously war certainly does not differentiate between one man and another, causing deafness indiscriminately. Silliness also stalks all classes, and although loud music usally affects mainly younger people, shooting without protection has sent unexpected people my way. Once, a Member of Parliament came with early hearing loss which was making it difficult for him to hear what was said in the House of Commons, and I advised that it might be a good idea to refrain from attending shooting parties.

"Impossible!" he shouted. He claimed that his political career depended on invitations to grouse or pheasant shooting parties at the great houses of England. Even my suggestion that he wear ear defenders was rejected out of hand.

"That would be sissy!" he said contemptuously. I thought that he must be very stupid indeed. Nevertheless, he ended up in the Cabinet so he must have known what he was about.

4.1.2.1 Assessment

Assessment of noise-induced damage should be straightforward as it depends on two main things. There must be evidence that the claimant had truly been subjected to excessive noise and an audiogram should show that there is indeed a hearing loss.

Hearing loss, by itself, is obviously not proof of noise exposure, even if the audiogram shows a typical pattern, as there are so many other causes of deafness and these patterns are very variable. All that the doctor, as an expert witness, can say is that noise is one of the possible causes in that particular case. It is for the claimant to prove, by arranging for sound measurements to be made, if necessary, that he had indeed been exposed to excessive noise.

Similarly, people who have been exposed to noise cannot ask for compensation if they have no hearing loss, as compensation is made for deafness but not for exposure alone.

Audiometrically, a drop in the hearing or "notch" at 4 kHz is typical of such damage (Figure 16) but that does not mean that other less typical graphs cannot also be the result of noise.

Many people suffer from both noise exposure at work and presbyacusis (hearing loss in old age), as by the time they claim compensation they have reached retirement age.

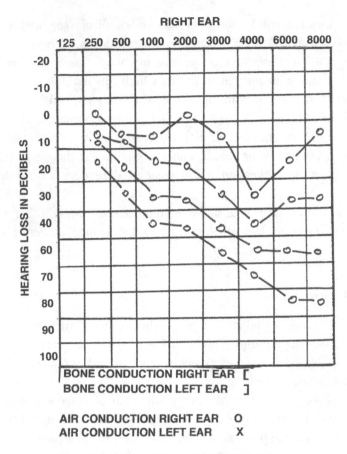

Figure 16. Audiograms in noise-induced hearing loss.

Hearing loss is often not identical in both ears as exposure is rarely the same on both sides. Rifle shooting is likely to deafen the left ear of a right-handed person as that is the one nearest to the explosion. Motorcyclists who have to listen to information by wearing a receiver in one ear and have it loud enough to override the background noise are all affected on one side. Nevertheless, sometimes the reason is not so obvious and it may simply be that one ear is more vulnerable than the other.

If a person who has been exposed to excessive noise suffers from a hearing loss, it remains for the defendant to prove an alternative explanation and it is unacceptable, within the limits of probability to suggest that there is an "unknown cause", without evidence of what it could be.

4.1.2.2 *Dangerous levels of sound*

Sound levels in the environment are measured by an instrument which consists of a microphone, an amplifier and a display which presents its recordings in decibels.

As we can make our measurements within a number of different ranges, the sound level meter also contains an attenuator to select among different ranges which are named A, B, C and D. We usually use the A range, and that is why noise levels are displayed as dB(A).

We know that sounds above 90 dB(A) can damage the sensory hair cells of the inner ear, but we are not confident about the safety of sounds that reach only 85 dB(A), and calculating exposure to noise is more complicated than mere numbers.

To express all the variable peaks and troughs over a lifetime's exposure we use a notional level which would be equivalent to a continuous sound during a particular time. We call this the Leq.

A notional Leq of 90 dB(A) is the equivalent to the same damage as exposure to 93 dB(A) for four hours or to 96 dB(A) for two hours and so on. Setting these standards has allowed people who have been deafened by noise to be compensated, but more importantly, have allowed us to protect personnel in the work place.

Four groups of measures are generally taken to do this. The first is to recognise which are the potentially dangerous areas. The second is to control the volume of noise by designing better machinery or simply by placing screens between the worker and the machine. Then we have to provide ear defenders in the form of ear plugs and ear muffs. The latter give a better attenuation but are not easy to wear over long periods especially if the worker also has to wear a protective visor. Finally many industries regularly test their employees so that the onset of even slight hearing loss will reveal those who are the most vulnerable.

4.1.2.3 *Compensation*

Although it had been known for a long time that excessive noise could damage workers' ears and it was referred to under different names such as "blacksmith's deafness" or "boilermakers' deafness", there was a certain informality about this. Even research which, as far back as the 1930s, had shown that those exposed to sound at 95–100 dB(A) were liable to lose their hearing tended to be looked upon as of mainly academic interest until the Second World War gave rise to much greater public awareness. A committee was set up to study the effects of noise. Its findings led to a Ministry of Labour publication in 1963 of a guide called *Noise and the Worker*, and it is from that date that a legal duty to protect workers arose. As a result, compensation may only be given for hearing loss incurred after that date.

I once gave evidence before a judge in the High Court, quoting from Bernardino Ramazzini, and since the lawyers seemed absorbed by the tale of that enlightened physician I thought I had made a great impression.

"That is all very interesting," the judge said finally, "and we are all very grateful for your information, but legally speaking, noise-induced hearing loss was not known before 1963!"

The first case to come before the English Courts was in 1971, generally referred to as "Berry" although it was the complex case of Berry vs Stone Manganese Marine.

Mr Berry had worked for 15 years as a propeller clipper, a very noisy occupation where he was subjected to levels of 115–120 dB(A), so he had become very deaf. The judge assessed the damages to £2,500 though Mr Berry only got half that due to the law of limitations, which meant that he could not be compensated for the early part of his exposure. I believe that all subsequent cases have been based on that figure, calculated for inflation since the fateful year of 1963, and whether the hearing loss was greater or less than that of Mr Berry, and to what degree.

In England most cases are dealt with in the same way as Common Law Actions, although servicemen can claim directly for hearing loss sustained while in the Armed Forces. There is also provision for industrial injuries compensation for those employed in certain prescribed occupations including those using drilling, pneumatic percussion tools and so on. Disablement benefits became payable from 1975.

4.1.2.4 *Other noises*

The 20th century has been a time of military forces so huge that the world had never seen or even imagined anything of the sort to be possible. The

French alone had put six million men under arms in 1939 and the Soviet and American armies were twice as large but it is unlikely, in an era of sophisticated technology, that whatever hostilities may come about, anything similar will happen in the 21st century and perhaps ever again.

Firearms, however, have not disappeared nor has the damage they cause to the ears. Ear protection is not now considered a sign of feebleness and, on the contrary, it is those who refuse to wear them who are considered inadequate.

The Army and the police always train with protective muffs and I have found that it is the instructors who are the most at risk, as even when they are not themselves firing, they are surrounded by those who are. Often, pistol practice takes place indoors and the resulting reverberation exacerbates the problem.

New and unexpected noises are always around us. Some years ago I was summoned to the maternity ward by the nurse in charge who demanded that I check one of the incubators in which premature babies were placed. I am no technician, and I knew nothing about incubators, but she literally forced my ear into the opening and I heard the most unpleasant cacophony.

"Is it right," she asked, "that our premature babies have to hear such an awful sound?"

We managed to demonstrate that although the levels were only around 85 dB(A) that was enough to damage the immature ears of the premature babies and that may have partly explained why such a high proportion were left with a hearing loss. When I look back at what I have done with my life I think that putting an end to that situation was one of the best things I ever did.

Recently, I was told that there had been a recurrence of deafness in these tiny babies in the region around Montpelier in France and that it had been traced to the introduction of helicopters to transport them to a purpose built and technically advanced unit. It had taken a while before it was realised that no provision had been made to protect the babies from the high noise levels of the engines.

Acoustic shock injury is another recent term which refers to acoustic incidents, particularly loud sounds emitted through headsets, which causes both stress and damage to the ear. The original descriptions have referred to incidents which occurred in call centres and were reported by Janice

Milhinch in Melbourne, Australia. There has been an expansion of work involving headsets in very recent times and this is likely to increase substantially in the years to come. There is no doubt that such injuries will become more frequent as the loudness we can expect amounts to a daily dose equivalent to 85 dB Leq or to peaks of sound of more than 120 dB SPL. Patients have described these unexpected sounds coming through the headphones as "shrieks", "howls", "screeches" and "squawks". This is not the result of an electric shock but Milhinch sees it rather as an emotional response to an unexpected loud sound. There is, however, also damage to the cells of the cochlea which may result in hearing loss and tinnitus.

4.1.2.5 *Psychological trauma*

I have been asked many times to say that irritating and unpleasant noises damage the hearing. This is because there is legal provision to protect people from physical injury to the ear, and if need be, to compensate them, while psychological trauma and stress are more difficult to handle. Indeed, we have not moved far from the Talmudic decision that such insults or provocations are not really the province of the earthly courts, presumably being best left to the heavenly ones.

Anyone who has lived with a teenager will be familiar with the anguish that the repetition, again and again, of the same loud refrains will cause. There are many other irritating noises such as the sound of trains or of cars travelling along main roads which damage the peace of mind without any evidence that the ears have been affected. While our technology cannot yet show images of our mood changes, the Freudian psychoanalyst, Bruno Bettelheim, believed that sounds that he found offensive, such as the music piped into elevators or shops, was an intrusion into his privacy. Those who move away from cities, seeking refuge in the countryside, are often disappointed by the noise of tractors and chainsaws (not to speak of the smell of manure).

In the year 2000 Villepointe, a suburb of Paris, undertook an extraordinary project in an attempt to deal with the noise created by a highway, using techniques only recently available and resolving the problem of noise in a truly novel approach.

Pneumatic tyre treads are set vibrating by the bumps in the road and the vibrations are transmitted to the whole tyre so that the walls produce the sounds we hear as the cars pass by. The air trapped between the rubber blocks of the treads is squeezed out through the grooves and, as the tyre adheres to the surface and then lifts up, it produces a "stick and snap" effect which is then amplified by the resonance of the tyre. In cars, the loudest sound has a frequency of 1,000 Hz; in trucks it is 600 Hz.

Armed with these facts, the suburb of Villepointe was able to add corrugations to the surface of their noisy road with such precision that, as the cars sped by, they produced a rather pleasant 28-note melody. Sadly, that imaginative solution failed as those who lived nearby claimed that the constant repetition of the same tune drove them mad and the road was re-asphalted two years later so it seems that only personal psychological resources can counter psychological stress.

The effect of traffic noise sometimes produces bizarre effects on nature as well on people. Researchers in Berlin, for instance, studied the songs of nightingales in the city. They measured the loudness of the birds' voices in streets, parks and woodland and found that they rose enormously in volume next to the Potsdammer Chaussee dual carriageway, where the birds had to sing at levels of 93 dB in order to be heard above the din of the rush hour. This was 14 dB above that in the quieter parts of Berlin, which means about five times as much in sound pressure terms, though the scientists did not say whether these birds suffered from laryngitis. Nightingales, of course, depend on making themselves heard in order to find a mate especially in the spring.

4.1.3 Hazardous drugs

Some drugs can damage the ear and affect both hearing and balance, and cause tinnitus. We call them *ototoxic* drugs and, although we should use them with care, they are often life saving.

The most commonly used ototoxic drug is aspirin. It is synthesised in laboratories as a white powder, hence its name, which comes from the Greek word for white, *aspro*. The active ingredient comes from the willow bark, which has served as a medicine in various forms as far back as mankind can remember. It may be the most useful drug ever, as it is an excellent painkiller and has an extraordinary capacity to reduce fevers. Today we know that it also thins the blood and helps reduce disease of the heart and clotting in blood vessels. In fact, hardly a year passes without the discovery of yet another beneficial effect of this useful substance. Millions of symptomless people take aspirin routinely every day and as a result mortality from these conditions has been considerably reduced. Although one of its side effects is that it can damage the inner ear, causing deafness and tinnitus, it does not do so in the recommended doses of 75–150mg, or even when the dosage is doubled or trebled to relieve pain.

Aspirin has a particularly beneficial effect in certain inflammatory conditions such as rheumatoid arthritis, but here the quantities necessary to achieve results over a longer term need to be high, and often tinnitus and deafness occur. However, the damage is reversible if the patient stops taking the high dosage as soon as symptoms such as buzzing in the ears appear.

The doctors and apothecaries of the past were, as always, on the look out for valuable new plants and they took particular interest in the bark of other trees though none surpassed the willow. In the 15th century, the Jesuits in Paraguay noticed that the native people used cinchona bark to treat fevers very effectively. It was even more useful than willow in the treatment of a malign, often fatal, tertiary fever which lasted three days and then recurred relentlessly. As that fever was generally believed to be caused by breathing in the bad air, or *mala aria* in Italian, which lay heavily over swamps, it was eventually named malaria. The extract from cinchona bark became known as quinine and its use allowed the extension of human habitation over large, previously uninhabitable, areas of the world. We know now, of course, that the "bad air" was actually the mosquito-borne malarial parasite and that it is destroyed by quinine. As with aspirin, quinine can cause damage to the ear but, like aspirin, the damage can be reversed if the drug is stopped as soon as buzzing is experienced. Malaria is so serious, however, that quinine treatment may need to be continued, despite the risk of deafness. Although there are other antimalarial drugs available they too have their own side effects and quinine remains an important part of the management of malaria, though not as a prophylactic.

Gin and tonic or gin and bitters were popular drinks among the colonials in malarial parts of world as an anti-malarial precaution. The alcohol in the blood stream may have weakened the parasite and tonic water contains quinine, the best anti-malaria medication available, which gave the bitter taste to tonic water. It is likely that quinine saved more lives than anything else until penicillin became available in the 1940s, although the latter did not help at all against malaria.

Tuberculosis, known in the past as consumption, was another major scourge which frequently affected the young, causing chronic ill health and even death. There was initially no specific treatment and all that could be done was to try to strengthen the body by rest and good food and, if they had the means, to live in places where the air was pure and unpolluted by the smoke of industrial cities.

Social collapse and malnutrition throughout Europe and Asia in the first half of the 20th century resulted in the rampant spread of tuberculosis during the two world wars and in their aftermath. The outcome would have been catastrophic if Selman Waksman and his associates had not discovered *streptomycin*. The discovery heralded the successful battle against tuberculosis. Streptomycin causes loss of balance as well as deafness, but it saved countless lives in its early days. Indeed, the same side effects are present with other powerful antibiotics like neomycine, gentamycine, and kanamycine, when taken by injection or by mouth.

Antibiotics such as these are also available in the form of ear drops but the literature that the manufacturers supply with them causes much anguish to those who read it. In order to protect themselves from litigation, they warn that there is a danger of deafness if they are used in an ear which has a perforated tympanic membrane. Such a consequence must be so rare that I doubt it is true, as I have never seen or heard of this ever happening to any of my patients, or to those of any surgeon that I know.

On the other hand the germs that cause many ear infections are so virulent and insensitive to every "safe" antibiotic that they may be life-threatening and can certainly put the hearing at risk. Treatment by drops containing gentamycine, neomycine and other ototoxic drugs is often essential, and putting such warnings against them seems to me to be an overreaction which can be harmful if it discourages the use of such drugs.

Some anti-cancer drugs such as cisplatinum also often cause some degree of hearing loss.

4.1.4 *Infections of the inner ear*

Infections of the inner ear can be due to bacteria or to viruses.

4.1.4.1 *Bacterial infections*

The inner ear is a self-contained, isolated structure, unlike the middle ear which, after all, communicates with the nose and is open to all sorts of germs every time we have a cold. The middle ear is able to tolerate frequent infection and survive intact but a germ which enters the inner ear spells doom as it can often cause total deafness and loss of balance.

Bacterial infection can reach the inner ear either by extension from the middle ear if it is not treated promptly and adequately or as a result of meningitis. That is why meningitis so often leads to profound deafness.

Treatment is based on large doses of the right antibiotic but by the time the infection has reached the inner ear there is very little chance of saving the hearing and we aim instead at saving the patient's life.

4.1.4.2 *Viral infection*

We often attribute sudden neurosensory hearing loss, sometimes associated with dizziness, to a viral infection, though we hardly ever have any proof.

That it does happen we can be certain as the hearing may occasionally be lost during an attack of mumps, itself a virus infection. We observe such a sudden loss of hearing from time to time also associated with a peculiar form of shingles which gives rise to vesicles around the ear and which we know is caused by a virus related to chicken pox as it resembles its virus in a more localised form.

There are antiviral drugs, but they are not effective once the hearing has been lost. Nevertheless, some comfort can be derived from the fact that that the viruses never seems to strike both ears.

4.1.5 *Vascular "accidents"*

We have no proof that vascular accidents exist at all and if they do we have no idea how often such a thing happens nor can we identify those in whom it has occurred. Arteries to the heart or the brain do get blocked, causing a heart attack or a stroke so it is not unreasonable to imagine that this can happen to the tiny artery which leads to the inner ear and cause sudden deafness. On the other hand we would expect that such events should be more common in older people who have diabetes and high blood pressure, and this is not the case. There is also no evidence that drugs which thin the blood or dilate the arteries have any effect whatsoever in relation to sudden deafness.

4.1.6 Immunological conditions

Occasionally we see patients who develop a neurosensory hearing loss in one ear associated with dizziness. The dizziness improves relatively quickly but the hearing loss persists and soon begins to affect the other ear. Very often there are symptoms and signs in other systems such as rashes, joint and muscle pains and eye changes, while blood tests suggest an immunological condition. This means that we have evidence that the body has turned against itself, as though it has developed an allergy to its own inner ear and tries to destroy it.

These disorders are very rare but very dangerous as the hearing may be lost altogether in both ears. On the other hand they do respond to treatment with massive doses of steroids which must be started as soon as possible. There is a problem, however, when we start reducing the dose, as the side effects of steroids are themselves relatively serious but if the hearing begins to deteriorate again, the specialist is placed in a dilemma. The dilemma is similar to when we turn to the same sort of powerful drugs after organ transplant operations to prevent rejection.

4.1.7 Injury of the inner ear

Most injuries today occur in road traffic accidents and those which result in a fracture through both the temporal bones are so serious that hearing loss is the least of the patient's concerns.

At the other extreme, mild concussion of the inner ear without a fracture is common and that may cause every degree of neurosensory hearing loss from a small dip or notch at 4 kHz, as in noise-induced damage, to total deafness.

Neurosensory hearing loss may be associated with a conductive loss as well, as the ossicular chain may have been disrupted. This conductive element can be repaired but it is important to appreciate how much of the hearing can be recovered by surgery before making a decision.

More serious injury, where a fracture extends into the inner ear, means total deafness on that side, and surgery has no place other than to repair a leak of cerebrospinal fluid which will not stop by itself or to free a facial nerve which has been crushed.

Tinnitus often accompanies the deafness though it tends to become less of a problem over two years or so in most cases. In others it becomes associated with depression and other psychological consequences.

All these injuries also involve loss of balance, but it is surprising how quickly most people recover through accommodation and adaptation.

Whiplash injury is now extremely common and can result in tinnitus and loss of balance, though hearing loss is very unlikely unless there has also been concussion.

4.1.8 Menière's disease

The symptoms of this disease are repeated attacks of vertigo, fluctuating deafness and tinnitus.

In the middle of the 19th century when Queen Victoria sat on the throne and Napoleon III ruled France, a French physician called Prosper Menière described, in a series of publications, a number of patients with a particular group of symptoms associated with the ear that seemed to occur regularly, pointing to a single disease. No one knew the cause of the illness; indeed we are not sure even now, and it is thus still called *Menière's disease*, despite the efforts of the usual iconoclasts to give it irrelevant and incongruous names from time to time.

Incidentally, Menière's family liked to style themselves "Ménière", with an acute accent as well and after his death they spelt it that way on his tomb, though it is simply "Meniere" on the family vault in the cemetery at Montmartre in Paris.

Although Menière was the first person to have realised that he was dealing with a specific disease different from other forms of vertigo or deafness, he was not the first to have described the symptoms, and I think that the saddest and most vivid evocation of the disease is that of the writer Jonathan Swift who suffered the condition from a young age.

> Deaf, giddy, helpless, left alone
> To all my Friends a Burthen grown,
> No more I hear my Church's Bell,
> Than if it rang out to my knell:
> At thunder now no more I start
> Than at the rumbling of a Cart;
> Nay, what's incredible, alack
> I hardly hear a Woman's Clack.

Menière's disease has three symptoms: vertigo, fluctuating hearing loss and tinnitus. Patients are often told that they have "Menière's" when they describe themselves as feeling dizzy, but it is wrong to diagnose so quickly unless the patient has all three symptoms.

Vertigo means attacks of dizziness producing a marked sense of rotation. Sometimes it is so severe that people are thrown to the floor. There is never, however, any loss of consciousness and if that does occur the illness cannot be Menière's disease. The dizzy attacks can last seconds, minutes, hours or even days when the patient is bed-ridden, and it is quite impossible to predict how often these episodes are likely to occur. They may be so frequent that life becomes impossible, or else years may go by without any trouble.

Associated with the vertigo is a fluctuating hearing loss which affects mainly the lower frequencies and although it tends to recover after each attack, there is a general downhill trend over the years. The deafness involves all the tones and deterioration occurs in sudden episodes rather than gradually.

Tinnitus is often described as sounding like "machinery" or, by the more imaginative, like "a sea shell held against your ear". It is often loudest at the onset of an attack when the patient also has a feeling of tension or fullness in the ear.

There are variants, of course, as with everything, and the oddest is called *L'Hermoyez's syndrome* after another Frenchman. In this variant, deafness heralds an episode and when the vertigo strikes the hearing improves. That is why it is also known as *"le vertige qui fait entendre"*, meaning the vertigo that makes one hear.

It is generally believed that Menière's disease is caused by an increase in the fluid pressure inside the inner ear and there is some evidence for that. It affects only one ear and I now believe that if the other is affected shortly after the first it is a very strong indication that it is not Menière's disease at all but one of those grim immunological conditions which leads inexorably to total deafness unless it is treated at once with massive doses of steroids.

The disease usually appears between the age of 40 and 60. There is no specific treatment for Menière's disease but as its evolution is so variable, every type of medication or change in life style has been tried both successfully and unsuccessfully.

There is no doubt that being of a calm disposition is more helpful that having neurotic tendencies, but psychotherapy has not found a place in the management of the symptoms even though it may contribute in other ways.

Advice on managing Menière's disease often involves changes to diet and lifestyle, which varies according to each generation's prejudices and beliefs. Coffee was once on the "prohibited" list, for reasons best known at the time even though it acts as a diuretic and helps to get rid of excess fluid. In fact, other diuretics were widely used as medication for Menière's disease in the hope that it would reduce fluid pressure in the inner ear. More generally, low salt diets are sometimes insisted upon; although this may be a good idea for those with hypertension, it is not a good suggestion for those who live in hot climates and lose a lot of salt through sweating. Likewise, red wine is recommended nowadays as part of a healthy diet.

Drugs which work well for sea-sickness are very useful in controlling an attack and help to calm the nerves in association with a few days' rest. The vast majority of sufferers manage to lead entirely normal social and professional lives despite the very disabling attacks that come from time to time; only a small number require surgery.

There are three operations that have found favour over the years. The first is based on inserting a small drain inside the skull allowing inner ear fluid to leak out when the pressure builds. Although technically difficult, it works well enough in my experience to be worth performing as a first step as it also helped preserve the hearing. When the symptoms recur frequently, making the patient's life impossible, and where the hearing is so poor that it is not worth preserving, labyrinthectomy should be considered. This is a destructive operation as the inner ear is irreversibly put out of action so any residual hearing is lost forever. The advantage is that it is easy to carry out and that the attacks of vertigo disappear permanently.

It is possible to cut the nerve of balance, the vestibular nerve, while preserving that of hearing so that the abnormal vertiginous sensations do not reach consciousness and in theory it appears to be the best option. In practice, however, it carries quite a large risk as it is an intracranial operation. Moreover, it does not arrest the deterioration of the hearing. Making the decision between the operations is delicate and difficult.

4.2 Disease of the Nerve

A viral infection of the nerve of hearing is so closely related to that of the inner ear that it is difficult to separate the two, if indeed they can be separated. Tumours inside the skull can press on the nerve and cause hearing loss.

4.2.1 *Acoustic neuroma*

The acoustic or auditory nerve is the eighth in the row of twelve cranial nerves which leave the brain and pass out of the base of the skull or cranium through a number of small holes. The first nerve is the one which transmits the sense of smell to the brain and the second cranial nerve carries vision. These emerge far from the acoustic nerve, which leaves the brain just behind the seventh, the facial nerve, which allows us to move the muscles of our face. These two nerves are so close together that a tumour of the one will affect the other.

The two nerves have hardly left the brain before they enter a canal in the temporal bone where the acoustic nerve splits up into two branches: one transmits hearing impulses from the cochlea of the inner ear and the other conveys the sensation of balance from the labyrinth. The facial nerve continues on its long voyage to the muscles of the face where it gives us our facial expression, our smiles and our ability to purse our lips to whistle or drink without spilling.

There is little space for this bundle of nerves to cross from the brain to the bony canal so that any tumour growing there will squeeze and damage them (see Figure 4). These are extremely rare but of those that do arise in that area, by far the most common are the *acoustic neuromas*.

These are not malignant in the sense that they do not spread throughout the body, and they also grow very slowly so that the danger they pose is entirely because of where they are sited as they will, in time, compress the brain itself.

The first symptom is usually a very gradual hearing loss in one ear. A gradual loss in both ears is not so worrying as it is very common simply from ageing, but when only one side is affected we become suspicious and we have to consider acoustic neuroma as a possibility.

Although balance is also affected, the very gradual nature of the loss of equilibrium means that it is rarely noticed. Sometimes the facial nerve shows very slight signs of weakness, though this symptom is by no means common.

There are variants, of course, and occasionally the presence of a tumour is heralded by tinnitus in one ear, dizziness or a sudden loss of hearing. Extremely rarely there may be tumours on both sides, but by and large it is the one-sided nature of auditory failure that makes us suspicious.

The presence of an acoustic neuroma, however tiny, can be demonstrated by an MRI scan which has replaced an array of other investigations. Usually, only 3% of suspicious cases turn out positive.

Surgical removal may decrease the hearing further, sometimes destroying it altogether. The purpose of the operation is to excise the tumour before it gets large enough to cause worse symptoms. It is not without risk as the facial nerve may be damaged, leading to temporary or even permanent paralysis of that side of the face.

As it grows so slowly in many patients, especially those who are older, many prefer to review the size of the tumour with a scan and committing to surgery only if the growth seems to be getting out of hand. On the contrary, there is a strong indication for earlier intervention for younger patients where the growth of the tumour is usually faster.

Surgery is done using microsurgery. The procedure aims to remove the tumour without damaging the facial nerve and, if possible, save the nerve of hearing. It requires special skills and even then it may be necessary to leave some tumour material behind.

Stereotactic radio-surgery is also sometimes used, either alone or after microsurgery, if some tumour material has had to be left behind. The procedure first locates the tumour exactly using three-dimensional coordinates and then points a beam of radiation very precisely at the site. This avoids damaging the surrounding tissues but it does not get rid of the tumour altogether. The aim is to stop it growing or to slow it down.

4.3 Brain Deafness

If those parts of the brain to which we owe our awareness of the sounds around us are damaged we are, in fact, deaf, even though the ears themselves and the auditory nerves are intact. Such damage can be caused by strokes, tumours or from severe injury.

Very rare conditions are not usually at the forefront of our thoughts — we tend to discount what is improbable unless it forces itself upon us — as I found when I was called upon to travel to the Persian Gulf to see a sheikh who had lost his hearing.

In preparation, I filled my pockets with different types of hearing aids. My plan was to test the hearing with my audiometer, and then try out the various aids as, all said and done, finding the right hearing air is mainly a question of trial and error. I was checking the batteries when the sheikh's son came to fetch me, swathed in white robes and carrying a cardboard shoe box filled with hearing aids of every size and type, from every country in the world. It turned out that many specialists had been there before me and my plan of action was a waste of time. The sheikh's son told me that his father had been struck by another vehicle, while travelling in a car along Baker Street, in London. He had survived, thanks to emergency brain surgery, but he was left quite deaf. Specialists had been sent by various governments, apparently anxious to ingratiate themselves with the oil-rich state. None had been able to help him.

"Have you brought some more hearing aids?" he asked, looking at me doubtfully as I stuffed them back into my pockets.

His father hated them, he explained, as the visiting doctors had forced him to put them on but the amplified sound drove him mad and the spoken words remained unintelligible.

When it was explained to him that I was not going to make him wear hearing aids, the poor sheikh kissed my hand and wept so I was not sure what do next.

When I tested him with the audiometer it was clear that the hearing loss was so slight that it was no surprise he could not stand amplification. On the other hand I knew that I had only tested his ability to hear pure tones, whereas his problem was not being able to understand speech so I asked his son to mouth a list of words without making a sound. The sheikh was able to lip-read them all perfectly but when the words were repeated out loud, the young man hiding his mouth, his father could understand nothing at all. Amplifying the speech made things so much worse that he pulled off the ear phones immediately.

The ears had hardly been affected and it was the parts of the brain which interpret what is heard that did not function. Making things louder was counterproductive as it confused the visual input from reading the lips with sounds which, to him, were meaningless.

Brain deafness is so rare that when it does happen it can be missed. The sheikh's case was special as visitors were received in a vast room called the *majlis* where each one brought a crowd of retainers with him, everybody clustering around the sheikh in a deafening hubbub. Once we had understood the problem, we placed a barrier beyond which only his personal friends were allowed to pass and speak to him quietly one at a time so that he could read their lips.

In these unusual cases communication can be reinstated in a roundabout way by encouraging a visual strategy, rather than hearing aids. I suspect that there is some element of brain deafness in many old people who may have a hearing loss as well, complicating the problems of ageing.

4.4 Born Deaf

One out of every thousand babies in the United Kingdom is born with a permanent hearing loss and an equal number become deaf in the first year of life. The figures vary to some extent because of the methods used to record the data, but they are similar in most countries of the same social level. In the United States, for instance, these cases are estimated at between 1 and 6 babies per 1,000.

Efforts are made to be as precise as possible so we know, among other things, how many children will need special help in education. The importance of identifying those babies who are born deaf has been recognised ever since it was realised that the possibility of acquiring speech was dependant on early teaching.

Often we never find out what has caused the deafness, but of those we do, about half have genetic causes while the rest are caused by many different factors.

Premature babies, babies born before 32 weeks or those who have a birth weight of less than 2.5 kg (5.5 pounds) have a greater chance of being deaf. This seems to be due to the coexistence of many risk factors.

Infection in babies is usually caused by what are known as the TORCH organisms. The organisms are toxoplasmosis, rubella, cytomegalovirus, herpes simplex virus 2. The "O" stands for "other", which includes chickenpox, HIV and syphilis. These can be diagnosed early, thanks to blood tests.

If the mother's blood group is Rhesus negative and the father's positive, a condition known as *Rhesus factor disease* may occur. This disease causes deafness as well as other abnormalities but it can be prevented by injections to the mother from 28 weeks.

As many as two thirds of babies can be a little jaundiced at birth, and this usually causes no problems. If jaundice becomes severe, the substance which gives the yellow colour, bilirubin (which is itself the breakdown product of red blood cells) can be toxic. Severe jaundice can result in deafness, together with other problems. Treatment with light usually solves the problem, as the blue rays in sunlight get rid of the bilirubin excess and only rare cases require more extreme treatment such as an exchange blood transfusion.

Certain drugs such as the antibiotic gentamycin can damage the hearing and if the mother is required to take it during pregnancy the foetus may suffer. The worst drug-damage in history was that due to thalidomide, a drug put on the market in Germany in 1957 as a drug which reduces tension and anxiety. Soon it was offered to pregnant women suffering from morning sickness and sold in many countries over the counter and without prescription. However, in 1961, Dr William McBride, an Australian obstetrician, made the connection between thalidomide and the malformations. By the early 1960s over 10,000 children had been born with severe malformations, mainly of the limbs and perhaps half of them did not survive. Some also had abnormalities of the outer and middle ear and were severely deaf. I operated on a number of them, trying at least to create an ear canal and restore enough hearing so that a hearing aid could be inserted. By 1961, when the drug was withdrawn in the United Kingdom we had 2,000 babies born with malformations. In West Germany, out of 2,540 cases, 262 suffered from total deafness and 628 had varying degrees of hearing loss.

In the United States, Dr Frances Oldham Kelsey, a new medical officer at the Food and Drug Administration, refused to licence the drug without further tests and thus saved thousands of children. Some pregnant women were still given thalidomide but I believe that only 20 babies were born with malformations. Dr Kelsey was decorated by President John F. Kennedy for his prudence.

Other causes of deafness in babies include birth injury and lack of oxygen. Both of these can cause other damage to babies.

Improved maternity units with adequate perinatal care, vaccination against rubella and other viruses has greatly diminished the risks to the baby, and the ability to offer genetic advice has also begun to make a difference.

4.4.1 *Genetics of deafness*

Farmers have known about selective breeding of both plants and animals for thousands of years so the knowledge about an offspring's inheritance of traits from their parents has been understood for a long time. Deafness has been known to be inherited for a long time.

In the middle of the 19th century, in what is now the Czech Republic, the Augustinian friar and science teacher, Gregor Mendel, was the first to carry out experiments interbreeding tall and short peas. It was only after he was long dead that he was recognised as the father of genetics, the whole process being called the Mendelian inheritance. During his lifetime, few knew about genetics; even Darwin never heard of him. Mendel did well for himself, however, becoming the abbot of his institution and founding the Austrian Meteorological Association. When he died in 1884, the famous composer Leoš Janáček played the organ at his funeral.

In his experiments, Mendel showed that there were discrete units of inheritance for particular traits which we now call *genes*. They are molecules located on long strands of DNA which twist into a double helix and are stored together as *chromosomes*. Our complement of genes is known as the *genome* and they act as the code to manufacture the various proteins that direct the structure and function of the body. If one or more genes, for one reason or another, has been changed, then an abnormality, such as deafness, may result and the change is called a *mutation*.

Every cell contain 46 stores of genes or chromosomes and we inherit 23 from each parent. One pair of these are the chromosomes which decide which sex we are and are known as X and Y. If there is a Y chromosome the individual is a male, so that all males have inherited a Y from the father as well as an X from the mother and are known as XY. Females are those who have inherited their father's X as well as their mother's and are therefore XX. When a gene that has changed is on one of the sex chromosomes we call the resulting abnormality *sex-linked*. The 22 other pairs of chromosomes are called *autosomes* and mutations of any of their genes are said to cause *autosomal genetic disorders*. Many are now being identified, mapped and cloned.

4.4.1.1 *Autosomal recessive disorders*

Not all genes are equally powerful as we may inherit a defective gene from the mother but the father's may compensate for the defect and as a result there is no apparent abnormality. These genes are called *recessive* since the changes do not have any effect. If two quite normal people who both have one defective gene have a child, the child may inherit the defective gene from both and suffer from an abnormality. That type of genetic disorder is called *autosomal recessive*. We are all carriers of one such recessive gene or another whether we know it or not. Specialists who give genetic advice can calculate the risks.

If, for instance, a person whose deafness is an autosomal recessive type marries someone with no deafness genes, none of the children will be deaf but they will all have a defective gene which may come out in later generations if they, in turn, find partners who have the same, hidden, recessive gene.

This is more likely to happen in cousin marriages and in isolated or tightly knit communities where deafness of autosomal recessive origin is most common.

I believe that 30 such genes for deafness have been mapped but the work is progressing so rapidly that there is always more. One of these is quite widespread and is called *Connexin 26* or sometimes *GJB2* and is located on chromosome 13.

4.4.1.2 *Autosomal dominant disorders*

Some changed genes cannot be compensated for by normal ones and anyone who inherits them will be affected though perhaps only partially.

An example of a dominant gene that causes deafness is the one that results in otosclerosis, although it is not necessarily inherited as mutations can happen spontaneously. It is said that 10% of genetic deafness is caused in this way.

At least 40 such genes have been identified.

4.4.1.3 *Syndromic genetic disorders affecting hearing*

Sometimes abnormal genes affect the hearing and other structures, in which case the disorders are called syndromes and are often named after the people who first described them, although as the genes which cause them and the way they operate become identified it is likely that the names will change. These syndromes can be dominant or recessive, autosomal or sex-linked and account for 30% of genetic disorders.

Alport's syndrome is linked to the X chromosome but as males have only one X they are particularly badly affected and usually suffer from kidney failure whereas women may have a normal X from the non-defective parent which will compensate to some extent for the defective one. As men were usually treated by kidney transplants I treated the hearing of a number of men from the Renal Unit at Guy's Hospital who had survived from their kidney failure and went on to have normal children of their own. Their sons, of course would not have inherited the defective X chromosome.

Usher syndrome which affects the eyes as well as the hearing is inherited as an autosomal recessive and is probably the result of mutations in any one of ten different genes.

Waardenburg's syndrome is inherited as an autosomal dominant and it must be relatively common as some estimates claim that 1 in 30 students in schools for the deaf of both sexes and all races have that syndrome. Those affected show pigmentary changes, the most frequent being a white forelock and heterochromia iridis which means that the irises of the eyes are of different colours.

Treacher–Collins syndrome shows craniofacial abnormalities of different degree and the deafness is conductive. Often the outer ear is small, rotated or even absent altogether while the eardrum and middle ear ossicles are malformed or have failed to develop normally. The cheekbones are often absent and the jaw is small. During my career I saw many such patients as this condition is often amenable to surgery.

There are other syndromes which occur rarely but now that we are so rapidly identifying the genes responsible for deafness and beginning even to learn which chemicals they are coded for and fail to produce, future progress and treatment may turn out to be quite remarkable.

4.4.2 Warped eugenics

Despite the good that came out of the discovery of genetics, there is an important lesson to be learnt from the fashion of eugenics. There are some things people do that should not be forgotten.

Francis Galton, who was Darwin's cousin, tried to turn the theories of evolution into a proactive approach towards human development. Undeniably well meaning, he referred to it as *eugenics*, which was to be a process of improving the genetic quality of the species by encouraging the reproduction of positive traits and discouraging that of negative ones. The concept was most popular among the educated and progressive minds of the time and was widely favoured in Europe and America in the early years of the 20th century.

It was based, however, on a scarcity of scientific knowledge about what genes were; even the existence of DNA was not yet known. If there was any controversy it was to do with what traits were so negative that they should be weeded out. As eugenics became popular among the ruling classes the question turned to what action could be taken by governments. The debate involved suggestions from benign advice about birth control to abortion and sterilisation. The argument was between persuasion and coercion.

When the Nazis came to power in Germany in 1933 a decision was made to eradicate what they deemed "inferior" from the gene pool: Jews and gypsies were segregated and they also legislated against homosexuals and disabled people. On 14 July 1933 the Law for the Prevention of Progeny with Hereditary Disease was enacted, forcing the sterilisation of the deaf, blind, malformed and the manic-depressives as well as what were deemed "promiscuous women". There was a legal appeals procedure, though that was hardly ever successful. Sterilisation courts were set up and forced abortions took place in pregnancies as advanced as six months. Deaf people were not allowed to get married and 16,000 deaf people are thought to have been sterilised in this way by the time the Second World War began, the youngest at age 9.

By 1939 the Action T4 euthanasia programme had emerged and killing centres were built, usually disguised as factories with chimneys so that the corpses could be burnt after gold teeth had been extracted. It is estimated that 275,000 German adults and children were murdered by gassing, starvation or lethal injection because they were disabled, their lives classified as "unworthy".

In order to identify disabled people, questionnaires were sent to physicians, social workers, welfare agencies, public health officials, hospitals, institutions and nursing homes and, on 18 August 1939, a decree compelled doctors and midwives to report infants and toddlers with disabilities and later children up to the age of 17 for extermination.

We now know that, because of the way genetics and sporadic mutations work, the Nazis would never have eliminated deafness from the German population no matter how many they killed. What started off as good intentions eventually led to forced sterilisation and soon to genocide.

Unintended consequences are remarkable in where they lead. After the war the West German authorities were so anxious to avoid a culture of reporting disabilities that when the drug thalidomide was introduced, they failed to register thousands of births with malformations, resulting in the association between the two not being made until many years later.

4.5 Tinnitus

Towards the end of 1876 the Czech composer Bedřich Smetana wrote a string quartet which he called *From My Life*. Two years earlier, in 1874, he had been aware of a rushing sound in his ears as well as abnormalities in the pitching of octaves and by October of that year he was deaf and overwhelmed by a piercing, whistling sound in his head.

An hour's work at a time was all he could manage and he found that it had become difficult for him to concentrate on composition. However, despite fits of depression and quarrels with his wife he felt compelled to carry on and he composed his quartet around the tinnitus. The last movement, in particular, suggests the haunting whistle which was making his life such a misery and ends with the first violin fiercely playing an edgy tremolando in a harmonic E. The first performance was given to a group of friends with Dvořák playing the viola.

Despite his trials, Smetana composed a three-act opera, two symphonic poems, two song cycles and the *Devil's Wall*, an opera that took him three years to finish. The string quartet No 2 in D minor was written about a year before his death in 1884 from the late stages of the syphilis which had caused his deafness. He was completely deaf by then but his mind was full of musical images as well as confusing and unexpected sounds which he described as a "whirlwind of music".

Another famous composer known to be severely deaf was Beethoven. He also suffered from tinnitus. Nevertheless he was able to compose some of his greatest works and though it is true, of course, that these people were entirely out of the ordinary, it seems that tinnitus, unlike an external noise can be set aside in some way. How this is done or indeed exactly where tinnitus originates remains a mystery.

This is not from lack of conjecture in the past or of concentrated research in the present as it has always attracted special interest because of its strange nature and the fact that it is not a "real" sound or even a hallucination.

Ancient Babylonian medical texts usually follow the format of: "If a man has…" and then go on to offer advice on the treatment.

These documents were written in cuneiform script on clay tablets many of which have survived and it is among them that we find:

> "If a man's ear speaks…"
> "If a man's ear sings…"
> "If a man's ear whispers…"

The treatment advised is usually an infusion poured into the ear and as these can differ according to the way the symptom is described it may be that they believed these were different conditions. They felt that most illnesses were caused by demons which had invaded and taken possession of the person and the ancient Egyptian doctors who were probably much influenced by their Babylonian colleagues referred to the "bewitched ear" in hieroglyph texts which may date from as far back as the construction of the pyramids.

Although some Greeks believed that tinnitus was the gods speaking in disembodied voices and it is possible that they confused it with the hallucinations of schizophrenics, most followed the philosophy of humors which suggested that disease was the result of an imbalance of the elements which constituted the body, dismissing the possibility of demons as irrational.

Although we now have access to so many more facts than our ancient ancestors had, we still do not know the cause of tinnitus.

Tinnitus is a symptom and not a disease and there is no one "cause" for tinnitus just as there is no single "cause" of headache. Both can be due to tension but can also, very rarely of course, be the symptom of an intracranial tumour. Every other condition imaginable which falls between such extremes may also result in headache, tinnitus or both.

The pitch and volume of tinnitus varies widely and my very first clinical publication recorded my attempts to correlate the pitch of the tinnitus with any ear disease that may be present. I did find some connection between the two but there were so many patients with no obvious disease that, in the long run, matching the pitch did not prove useful.

Any disease of the outer, middle or inner ear or nerve can cause tinnitus and the characteristics of the symptom are unlikely to give much indication as to the underlying cause. If there is any obvious abnormality or hearing loss, as in the case of noise exposure, Menière's disease, otosclerosis or even wax then it is reasonable to associate the two. Tinnitus is also more common as we get older and our hearing deteriorates.

Pulsatile tinnitus which follows the heart beat is not uncommon and like the other types of tinnitus rarely represents anything specific but very occasionally a vascular tumour presents in this way. This will show in an MRI scan.

Tumours as a cause of tinnitus should be suspected if it affects only one ear and should be excluded by a scan too. When tinnitus is in both ears or "in the head" a tumour is so unlikely that unless there are other suspicious indications it does not warrant investigation.

Another unusual type of tinnitus is a clicking sound in the ear. This is different and has to do with the opening and shutting of the Eustachian tube. We can occasionally see a sort of muscular tick as the soft palate jerks in time with the click which can even be heard if we hold an ear close to the patient's. The muscles of the palate pull the tube open periodically making the clicking sound.

Tinnitus is sometimes present in noise-induced hearing loss and is commonly found as a result of head injury as well as of whiplash. For the purpose of compensation it is usually classified as slight, moderate or severe though this seems to be decided on the whim of the examiner and on the persuasiveness of the client as the severity of tinnitus is not clinically measurable.

A few patients who suffer from depression say that that tinnitus can be an indication of deterioration and be very disturbing though it gets better as recovery sets in.

As an interesting aside, I was perplexed when I went through my cases and found that among the women over 50 who had come to me complaining of tinnitus and who had no obvious cause, many had a daughter who was going through a divorce, though it did not apply to the men who had tinnitus or to divorcing sons. We can only speculate as to what this means.

Where the tinnitus actually starts is obscure, but Dr Abraham Shulman in New York showed me PET (positron emission tomography) scans which can look at parts of the brain and it seemed to me that there is every likelihood that even if the initial damage was in the ear, the symptom itself is the result of activity in the brain.

It is hardly surprising that with so little known about the mechanism of tinnitus the treatment also leaves a lot to be desired. This does not mean that no treatment is offered as, on the contrary, the different approaches are countless and every physician has his own favourite whether it works or not.

At one conference on tinnitus every doctor who stood up seemed to present a different treatment. Psychotherapy was apparently successful in some hands while others claimed recovery with antidepressants. Some had been using electrical stimulation and some reported success with sound stimulation. The latter has been commercialised in the form of a tinnitus masker that looks like a hearing aid and produces a white noise. It has proven helpful to many patients and it seems that an external sound which drowns the internal one is beneficial, though some have told me that they prefer to listen to Mozart especially in the loneliness and silence of the night. One man rather bizarrely switches his shortwave radio to a station speaking a language he cannot understand as after a while he finds that it eases the tinnitus. Listening to a language with which he is familiar does not help him sleep and he tells me he favours a Bulgarian station. Some doctors have reported that ginkgo biloba is effective in Germany while in England it rarely seems to help.

One physician was asked to tie up all these suggestions and review the treatment. He chose to quote the 12th century philosopher and physician, Maimonides, who had been asked if it was permissible to use spells when treating patients on the Sabbath. At that time spells and amulets were widely employed by doctors, but they were uneasy about using magic on the Sabbath. The sage, a rationalist, replied by ridiculing belief in magic altogether but he nevertheless ended by saying: "…if you think an amulet or a spell or whatever rubbish can help your patient then use it by all means, even on the Sabbath".

As our own contemporary sage was greeted with silence he added: "I suppose we are entitled to fool our patients if we think it will help them but whatever we do please let us not fool ourselves."

Tinnitus occurs in a number of conditions and follows many injuries of the head and neck, but we can only speculate on the mechanism that sets it up. We have no remedy that cures it but we do have many treatments that help people to live with it.

Part III

Communication

We can communicate using our visual, olfactory and tactile senses as well as hearing. Language, the basis of communication, involves sound when it is expressed as speech, but if sound is not used or not available we still have writing and gesture. Music is a form of communication that uses sound, and poetry too has its own particularity.

We know what we mean by communication but when we start to think about it unexpected aspects to come to mind.

For instance do we communicate by smell as animals do? We know that male dogs identify their territory in that way and that the females will express their sexual receptivity through odour. There is uncertainty as to whether humans also use such chemical signals to communicate subconsciously.

We communicate visually through signs and symbols. Arrows indicating direction have been used before writing was invented and the array of wordless traffic signs is part of our daily life.

Our ancestors learnt to express what they had to say in pictures. To indicate "man" they drew a man. For ease and speed the drawings became more symbolic than realistic, line drawings rather than portraits (Figure 17). These, in time, evolved into true writing as complex concepts

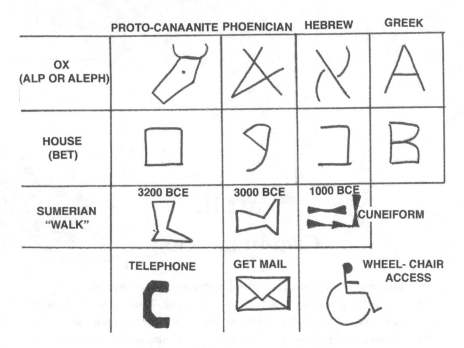

Figure 17. Pictograms become symbols.

had to be expressed and we find this in Babylonian cuneiform, Egyptian hieroglyphs and Chinese pictograms which are still in use now by the major part of the world population. The great advantage of picture writing is that it can be read by people who speak any language as a drawing or a symbol for "house" means a house whether we say it in German or French or English. Indeed we use such symbols to indicate men or women's toilets all over the world and we hope that they are usually understood (Figure 18)!

On the other hand, drawings can be cumbersome so some of the pictures started to represent sounds rather than concepts. They often had to be used to represent names or titles which were sounds rather than actions or ideas and so a phonetic element was introduced. When pictures represent sounds rather than concepts we can call them "phonograms". The Egyptian system of hieroglyphs contained both, which makes it very difficult for us to understand.

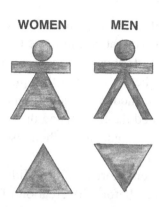

Figure 18. Signs for "Men" and "Women".

The first alphabets (a word which comes from *aleph-bet* or "A-B" of the early Semitic writing which survives in today's Hebrew and Arabic scripts) only indicated the consonants, though dots were later added to convey vowel sounds. When the Greeks copied it they introduced signs to represent specific vowels and in that form the alphabet was passed on to us.

Although our present writing, as a tool for communicating, can be understood without using speech, it remains a system of signs based on consonant and vowel sounds and not of symbols.

Among the various senses used in communication (smell, sight and touch), sound is one of the most important, although it does not necessarily involve language. A male song bird sings to outline his territory and to attract a female partner. That is communication but it is not language as it is automatic, each stimulus inducing only a pre-ordained response. In fact a female bird does not sing at all unless she is injected with the male hormone testosterone; when that happens, she sings automatically.

The development of sound communication into language is something else again. It seems not to have existed before the evolution of man, possibly around 200,000 years ago, and it may be seen as his most important invention. Indeed we have always been aware of its defining place but there has been great uncertainty as to how it reached mankind in the form that we know it.

A sensible place to start is the Bible. According to Genesis, in the beginning "was the word." God appears to have initiated the universe by the use of language, and later when Adam was created, the animals are shown to him one by one so that he can name them. The meaning of this story is remarkable, if mysterious, and the sages of the past spent much time discussing what lies behind it. To us the opinions of these sages, who did not have access to our modern research tools, are especially interesting. After all, they explored the mind using the mind alone and if we are able to make the effort to understand their use of metaphor it might provide us with an extra insight.

According to the ancient stories of the Midrash, the naming of the animals, which took place before the creation of Eve, upset the angels as God had told them that man's intellect would be superior to theirs. To prove the point he had asked them to name the animals initially, but they had been incapable of doing so. The sages suggested that the angels were designed to accomplish single missions and were unable to comprehend characteristics outside their own. Man on the other hand had the characteristics of the whole of creation and was therefore able to comprehend nature and to give it a name. It was he who called himself Adam as he was conscious of both his earthly origin and destiny; in Hebrew, earth is *adamah*.

When asked to name God, Adam calls him *Adonai* which simply means "Lord" and the true name remains a mystery. In fact it may not exist at all in a form that Adam and humanity can perceive.

In the 12th century an extraordinary mystical current that saw creation itself as a linguistic phenomenon developed among the rabbis of Spain. Under the name of *kabala* or "tradition" it was to have an important effect on the Christians as well as the Jews as a technique of interpretation of sacred texts.

According to the Kabalists there was a primordial Torah or Books of the Law before the known ones. It was not written in letters at all but in the form of black flames on white fire. It was a thought process, an emanation of the godhead, which only later became words.

It seems that the Kabalists had developed the concept that if we are to understand language as we express it and use it as a tool for communication we must understand also that it is preceded by an "inner language" which is a thought process.

They had understood that every human being is born with the capacity to know the whole of nature, the difference between an animate and an inanimate object, between a plant and an animal, between man and the rest of the animal kingdom even before he can name them in words.

On the other hand if every baby is born with the same inner language how is it that so many linguistic groups have developed along their own paths? Again thinkers have set their minds to this problem from the ancients to Noam Chomsky in our own time.

The Bible gives conflicting stories on the development of the various languages as on the one hand we are told in Genesis 11 that after the flood the residue of humanity had only one language which is understood to represent a degree of harmony among men.

It is when they decided on the construction of the Tower of Babel that linguistic history changed for ever. It seems that they had made an unwise attempt to reach the heavens. Some said, again according to Midrashic writings, that they were actually planning to attack the celestial regions with bows and arrows. The Lord thought, "Let us go down and confound their language that they may not understand one another's speech." And that was how the multitude of languages was born and, presumably as a result, strife among men.

On the other hand Genesis 10 tells a different story. When they had recovered from the Flood, Noah's three sons, Shem, Ham and Japheth and their descendants went their separate ways scattering and diffusing throughout the world: "Everyone after his tongue, after their families, in their nations."

No doubt the story of the Tower of Babel is the more exciting and inspires the imagination as it is also associated with morality and the sense of punishment.

Naturally there has been great interest throughout the centuries as to what was the first language. Herodotus wrote in his *Histories* that the Pharaoh Psammeticus had two newly born boys given to a shepherd who had been instructed not to speak to them at all. The purpose of this experiment was to see in what language they would speak spontaneously. Herodotus reported that that the boys' first words were "Becos! Becos!" which the shepherd did not understand but which apparently means bread in Phrygian, a language now dead. Thus, Herodotus concluded that the first language must be Phrygian.

This pagan assumption was questioned as Christianity spread across the Roman world and it was generally accepted that the first language must have been Hebrew as that was considered to be the language of the Bible and of Adam.

A number of kings are reported to have tried to repeat the Pharaoh's experiment, the last of which seems to have been King James I of England but the children mostly died in these conditions of deprivation or perhaps drifted away. At any rate no conclusion was reached.

Chapter 5

Language

We can have language without speech as a deaf person may express it by gesture. To not have the capacity for language is quite different from lack of speech as it separates us from our fellow men.

5.1 The God with No Mouth

Petra, in Jordan, not far from the port of Aqaba, is an ancient city carved into the red rock accessible through a narrow pass only on foot or on horseback.

Although its inhabitants were cave dwellers, the doorways of their buildings, openings in the cliff wall, are surrounded by the most elaborate carved pillars, capitals and reliefs and the interiors, cut deep into the rock form grandiose halls and numerous rooms decorated in a manner comparable to any in the Roman world.

Indeed, the Nabateans, as that was their name, were part of a wide trading civilisation with towns scattered around oases all over that desert region, connected by means of an extensive network of caravan routes.

Although they were masters of communication, the stretched-out pathways that held them together remained ephemeral, notions in the minds of the camel drivers who were guided by the stars or the occasional human artefact. Yet they proved strangely robust, lasting for centuries with little in the way of maps or instructions written down.

Among all the carvings that have survived are the features of their god, Elath, who is depicted with no mouth at all or occasionally with a tiny one, a dot at most (Figure 19).

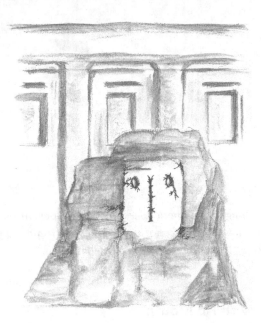

Figure 19. Elath, the god with no mouth.

A god without a mouth does not give orders or issue commandments regarding moral or social behaviour. He observes, certainly, through his big round eyes and we have to assume that he listens even though we cannot see his ears as he is only shown on a flat surface looking straight at us.

He is always depicted in this simplistic form even though the Nabateans could sculpt in the most sophisticated classical fashion so it must have meant something for them to want to represent him only in this manner.

A listening god in our time of psychotherapy is quite acceptable even if he does not speak or tell us what to do. After all we should work that out by ourselves while someone or something listens as we express our emotions and our fears.

5.2 An Inner Language

Even if we do not speak a particular language we can understand many international symbols such as discussed earlier, for example the difference between men's and women's toilets or traffic signs. We can get quite far in foreign countries simply using gestures, pointing to our mouths if we are hungry or indicating the need to drink or to sleep.

This suggests that we have a shared "inner language". We share it also with quite small children who may not understand the words we are saying but who can demonstrate they have already acquired our inner language. A cup will be brought to the mouth for instance or a brush to the hair showing they have learnt what these things are for, even before they have learnt their names.

It is a great comfort when assessing a child too young to have developed speech, to see it put a spoon to its mouth, pretending to eat. For the child, it is great fun when it places a tiny chair in front of a toy table and sits a doll on it. In fact, it is not just fun, as it shows that the child has grasped that these little objects, the toys, are actually symbols representing real ones.

In these tests, there is always one complaining mother who claims that her child was not "properly" tested but that "the specialist just played with the child". It's clear from the complaints that she has not understood that the capacity for symbolic play of this type indicates that her child has acquired inner language.

Even more comforting is the evidence that our child not only wants but needs to communicate.

We can express our inner language emotionally by music, using the forms which the composer has provided us with and we can reinforce the meaning of our words by putting them into songs or poetry.

We can emphasise what we mean by gesture and this may be an integral part of many spoken languages. If we cannot hear at all then we have to rely entirely on gesture but it is hearing and speech that we use to communicate most of the time.

I remember reading an article in the *International Herald Tribune* on mobile telephones, written by a journalist based in Hong Kong. He pointed out the availability of this form of communication to millions, shortly billions, of people but what struck me most was reading that if he needed to punish his teenage daughter he would ban her from using her telephone.

In a sense it was like sending her upstairs to her room, a common punishment in the past, cutting her off from communication with the world of people around her. A terrible punishment for the girl, even though she would still have access to books and perhaps television.

The punishment was not being cut off from news and information but being prevented from expressing herself by speech, giving her views to her friends, the verbal give and take of life known as "gossip".

5.3 Wild Children

We have accepted over the centuries that language is an innate attribute of human beings and that every child is born with the potential to communicate and that it is part of a more general capacity to recognise the difference between animate creatures and inanimate objects and also of the ability and need to communicate with others.

It is also likely that the inborn potential to put things together, to imagine and make complex tools or, in the young child, to put together bricks to make a tower, uses the same brain functions that can put words together and turn thoughts into sentences.

We have found that this potential is the same in all children whatever their culture, be it French or Japanese, Kalahari Bushmen or Australian Aborigine. Whether they are able to turn language into speech is another thing altogether. That if a child hears French words it will speak French and not Japanese is obvious. It should be equally obvious that if a child is deaf and cannot hear words at all it will not be able to reproduce words and will not speak. That is why we are so anxious to make use of any hearing that a deaf child may still have by amplification with hearing aids as soon as possible.

This makes us curious as to what would happen if a normally hearing child were deprived of contact with speech, but the rather brutal attempts by ancient kings to willfully deprive children in order to see what happens have not given us any information. The anecdotal evidence we have tells of what they did but not the result so we can only assume that either the children died or the kings forgot about it and their experiments were abandoned. One way or another they "failed".

Failure probably meant that the children simply failed to develop any speech at all rather than utter the "original" human language.

On the other hand there are some children who have, for one reason or another, survived alone in the wild and have never been exposed to any human speech.

These cases are very rare but have led to so much excitement that they have often been well documented. Perhaps humanity feels rather near the "wild" state and is conscious of civilisation being only a thin veneer, so that curiosity as to what the "real" man is has always attracted much attention. Maybe the popularity of psychoanalysis, both Freudian with its interest in early childhood and Jungian with its consideration of archetypes, stems from the same impulse.

Descriptions of wild or feral children as they are also known, traditionally start with Romulus and Remus, the abandoned twins who were rescued and fed by a she-wolf, *lupa* in Latin, and then went on to found the city of Rome.

The story is mythological and may also misrepresent the facts, as the word *lupa* was used by the Romans as a word for prostitute. Those who have visited the ruins of the brothel in Pompeii may remember that it was called the *luparium* or "wolf's den" and the twins may just have been abandoned babies brought up by a prostitute!

Although there have been frequent tales of lost children they are mostly anecdotal and it is only in 1726 that we find the first proper record. It is an extraordinary one and he was studied in an unexpected place as the wild boy came to live in St James' Palace and then Leicester House, as a curios of the royal family.

George I was the King of Hanover and had come over to London to become the King of England only quite late in life. The king was visiting Hanover when he was told that a boy had been caught in the forest roaming wild, living off plants and nuts. He was thought to be between 12 and 15 years old, naked and completely speechless.

The King asked to see him right away and, as he grew fond of the boy, eventually had him brought to St James' Palace in London. The aristocracy, the ministers and ambassadors were all invited to come and see him.

The wild boy fascinated Princess Caroline, wife of the heir to the throne, and she insisted on taking him to her own palace, Leicester House, which stood where Leicester Square is now. At first King George tried to resist her demands as he was a rather shy and reticent person and he had come to enjoy the effect that the totally uninhibited boy had on his rather boring court.

Interest in the wild state gripped everyone and it was said that some of the ladies of the court were more interested in the form that freedom of sexual behaviour would take, so that when the wild boy tried to kiss and fondle Robert Walpole's (the then Prime Minister) daughter it caused great amusement. Philosophical and political discussion, however, centred on the degree of control by church, state or even good manners that was necessary to lead to the happiness which was just beginning to be recognised as a human need if not yet a human right.

Jonathan Swift had made the trip from Ireland to the Princess's court, an invitation that he had previously declined. His book "Gulliver's Travels" had made him famous and his arrival must have been a feather in Princess Caroline's cap as she was desperate to surround herself with interesting people. The opportunity to see the wild boy attracted Swift and he was introduced by his friends the poet Alexander Pope and the physician Dr John Arbuthnot, to whose care the boy was entrusted and who named him Peter.

Although the doctor taught Peter some social graces in the sense that he learnt to bow when greeting people which indicates understanding of some aspects of language, he never learnt to speak.

Many who had observed the wild boy, and many who had not, wrote profusely about him in books, articles and pamphlets though none of them saw any interest in describing the methods used by Dr Arbuthnot in attempting to teach him how to speak and he himself did not do so.

Daniel Defoe was very interested in Peter. His own novel, *Robinson Crusoe*, with its study of Robinson Crusoe's relationship with Man Friday, is even now one of the greatest studies of loneliness and separation. But Defoe had other vested interests, as his daughter Sophia was being courted by Henry Baker who was a teacher of the deaf and dumb. Defoe knew a great deal of Baker's techniques for teaching lip-reading and speech to the deaf and he refers to it in a pamphlet, *Mere Nature Delineated or a Body Without a Soul* which he published in 1726, priced at one shilling and sixpence.

He points out a paradox as Defoe is quite sure that the soul is dependent on language:

"Words are to us the Medium of thought. We cannot conceive of things but by their names."

And later:

"All our passions and affections are acted in words and we have no other way for it."

On the other hand he tells of a deaf family in which only one child, a girl, could hear. The family communicated by gesture, which Defoe called "finger language", and the girl never learnt to speak. The fact that she could hear perfectly well was only discovered when she was 14. Despite much effort she never managed to speak properly.

Defoe seems to have understood that language and therefore the soul and humanity, can be expressed in the form of gesture but there still appears to be confusion about the difference between speech and language.

Not long after Peter had been found and his fame had spread throughout Europe, especially among the thinkers of the Enlightenment, a wild girl aged about ten was caught lurking in the woods near Songi on the River Marne in France and was taken to the Vicomte d'Epinoy. She had been living like a wild beast and had killed a dog in a single blow using a stick. She was finally captured by shepherds who enticed her down from a tree with food like any animal. She was given the name Memmie le Blanc.

Yet there was a difference from Peter, the wild boy, in that she was not naked, even though her clothes were rags. She also wore a necklace and had a pouch fixed around her waist in which she carried things including a small knife engraved with strange writing no one could read. This suggested that she must have had sort of early human contact, presumably including the use of speech even though there it may not have been French.

She could not speak a word, but gradually and painfully learnt French when her care was taken over by nuns under the protection of the Queen of France and her mother the Queen of Poland. Her capacity to learn to speak probably confirmed that the potential for speech was likely to have been established early on in her life, even though very briefly.

Her case drew the attention of Monsieur de la Condamine, one of the most famous scientists in France, who had just returned from a highly publicised expedition to the Amazon.

De la Condamine was a brilliant sceptic who had spent much time with the Indians while mapping the Amazon River and had formed a rather cynical view of them. Unlike the *"Philosophes"* of the enlightenment, he had little admiration for savages and had no illusion regarding the brutality of primitive life.

This was the opposite of Jean-Jacques Rousseau who was to publish his *Discourse on the Origins of Inequality*. It was from there that the concept of the "Noble Savage" and a certain nostalgia for the primitive state, its simplicity and its dignity had swept over the European educated classes. Needless to say, unlike de la Condamine, Rousseau himself had never met a savage, noble or otherwise, and it had all come out of his head.

De la Condamine befriended Memmie and helped her establish herself in Paris where she was supported by the Duke of Orleans until his death. After that she maintained herself modestly by making artificial flowers and selling copies of her biography by a Madame Hecquet, published in 1755 *Histoire d'Une Jeune Fille Sauvage Trouvée dans les Bois a l'Age de Dix Ans*.

De la Condamine took a Scottish lawyer, Lord Monboddo, to meet Memmie so that Monboddo could go over her story patiently and write it all down. Lord Monboddo had also visited Peter, who was by then at a happy old age, living with a farming family, unable to say anything other than a few syllables, though he enjoyed music and liked to sing wordless tunes.

The origins of Memmie remain obscure, but it is likely that she was born in a country other than France and taken by slavers at the age of about seven. Escaping from a shipwreck together with a black girl, she found herself in France. With the death of the other girl she reverted to savagery and completely forgot the words she knew.

Despite Lord Monboddo's assiduous note-taking and his previous meeting with Peter, he does not seem to have made the important distinction between Memmie and the Wild Boy.

Whereas Peter, who had apparently never learnt to speak and was unable ever to acquire speech, Memmie was able to learn French perfectly well even though that was certainly not her original forgotten language. She is likely to have spoken as a small child but forgotten the language when she lived in isolation.

It seems from the cases of these two children that speech must be acquired in the early years, but the language they learn is not important. This understanding has become the basis of the modern approach to teaching deaf children.

Long after Peter and Memmie had died, as well as Monsieur de la Condamine, France was to drag the world through momentous events.

Jean-Jacques Rousseau's thoughts on the origins of inequality and the Noble Savage, like those of Voltaire's *Ingenu* who had observed the sophisticated, class-ridden European society, had helped to put in motion the historic events of 1789 when Parisian crowds burnt down the Bastille. There were no inmates in that ancient prison but its destruction had and indeed still has enormous symbolic meaning.

In the following years the Revolution turned into a bloodbath and was soon replaced by a military dictatorship, only for the General, Napoleon Bonaparte, to proclaim himself Emperor.

It was then that another naked child seen running at great speed in the woods in the department of Aveyron was captured. He was handed over to Monsieur Boneterre, a professor of natural history who said that this was a wild boy and should be studied so as to understand the essential nature of man.

The revolution had set down the *Droits de l'Homme* or the "Rights of Man" without defining what the essence of humanity was and the boy, untainted by religion or society, he believed, was truly Rousseau's Noble Savage himself.

As he could not speak and seemed not to notice conversations around him he was at first thought to be deaf and was sent to the school for deaf mutes founded by the Abbé de l'Epee, and which was then run by the Abbé Sicard.

The best-known physician of the time in Paris was Phillipe Pinel, a most humane doctor who had removed the shackles from the insane in the lunatic asylum of the *Hôpital Bicêtre*. He had been asked to assess the boy but did not agree with Bonneterre and thought that he was simply an abandoned mentally retarded child.

Pinel felt that the boy's inability to relate to people, to experience or show affection or other types of social contact such as gratitude, meant that the prognosis was very poor. This, in his opinion, was certainly no Noble Savage.

In today's jargon I suppose he would have been termed part of the "Autistic Spectrum"

While at the Institute for Deaf–Mutes the boy was visited by Jean Marc Gaspard Itard, a young doctor who was earning extra money doing clinics at the institute while writing his thesis. Bright and ambitious, he was anxious to take on any challenge. Himself a pupil of Pinel, his enthusiasm and persistence was such that he managed to get himself appointed Resident Physician at the Institute and was put in charge of the wild boy of Aveyron.

The story of the education of Victor, the name the boy was given, was made into a film, *L'Enfant Sauvage* by François Truffault based on the detailed book that Itard himself had published.

Itard's efforts were successful to some extent, as Victor did form a relationship with him as well as with his housekeeper Madame Guercin and was able to indicate his needs by gesture such as offering his wooden bowl if he wanted milk.

He was never able to speak.

When I read Itard's account I tended to agree with Pinel that Victor was a child with a serious developmental disorder abandoned by parents who could not cope.

There have been a number of reports through time in India of abandoned children reportedly found in wolves' dens or living with wolf-packs. Such reports inspired the story of Mowgli in Rudyard Kipling's *The Jungle Book* and although the reports have enriched our imagination, most are unlikely to be true. The best documented case is that of Kamala and Amala, two little girls who were found in India near Midnapore and appeared to have been nurtured by wolves. They were found by a missionary, the Reverend J.A.L Singh, who took them to his orphanage in 1920.

It was not unusual in India for unwanted children, especially girls, to be exposed at birth and, although this is a unique case, it is well documented and photographed, suggesting that it is not impossible for children to be suckled by a she-wolf.

Although they had the same inability to relate to other people that we associate with autism, they were closely attached to each other and when Amala died of a gastrointestinal infection, Kamala was grief stricken.

It took much patience as well as kindness from Mrs Singh who often used physical contact by massage, before she managed to attach the girl to her. She began to understand the meaning of a few words and could communicate by gesture, but after eight years Kamala died too. Just like other children who had been isolated from human contact in their early years, she never spoke.

***

Can anything be learnt from these wild or feral children?

At the time of the Enlightenment many believed that studying these cases would confirm Rousseau's fantasies that the basic nature of humans still in a state of primitive savagery was something beautiful and noble. It was believed that the essential equality of all men had been corrupted by what we call civilisation. On the other hand, de la Condamine who had actually met savages in the Amazon had returned with a sceptical view, and supported science, morality and philosophy rather than any imagined innate feral nobility.

Everyone concerned with discovering the essence of man had no doubt that language was its most important aspect. Although they recognised that gesture was also a sort of language, they were unable to distinguish clearly between language and speech, its vocal expression.

Itard himself had been influenced by Étienne Bonnot de Condillac, a philosopher concerned with the development of identity and consciousness of the self, which could only be expressed as language, and presumably only existed when language came to exist. According to de Condillac, words came into being in response to needs and wants, and as these included the need to form bonds, names had to evolve.

Itard supposed that with the recognition of names and the understanding of relationships, sympathy also must come and he made that concept the core of his teaching of Victor.

Philosophising about the self and identity has continued, of course, but with the arrival of psychoanalysis in the 20th century people were able to delve into themselves. This proved a most attractive proposition, easily available, and it ceased to be necessary to wait for the appearance of a wild child to investigate the essence of mankind. The study of language itself, in the form linguistics and semiotics, became better organised and scientific and interest turned in that direction too.

The social sciences became less concerned with inequality as politics and economics took over that aspect. Instead it was deprivation and abuse and their effect on human development that began to attract attention. For these reasons, when the modern equivalent of a neglected child turned up in Temple City, Los Angeles, in the 1970s she caused enormous excitement.

She was an appallingly abused child who had reached the age of 13 locked up in a room with minimal exposure to language from her mother while her father barked at her like a dog.

The press, of course, took a great interest in the story and the experts were anxious to see how new understanding and theories regarding child care and rehabilitation from abuse would work out.

She was taught intensely and learnt to speak to some extent; like Memmie she had heard some human speech.

5.4 The Critical Period

From the evidence we have of these wild children we can draw only one conclusion: those who are not exposed to speech in early life fail to develop it. This observation corresponds with the concept of a critical period in the child's development when language is acquired and is expressed as speech. If that period is by-passed it is a great deal more difficult, often impossible, to acquire speech later.

This immediately poses another question. When does the critical period end? Or put another way, at what age have we missed our chance to teach a deprived child how to speak? This is of paramount importance to those who have to manage and educate the deaf child, and it was highlighted to me as a result of an unexpected experience.

In 1973 important political changes took place in the Middle East and the oil-producing countries suddenly increased their prices of oil. Under the chairmanship of the colourful Sheikh Yamani we regularly saw the leaders on television at meetings of the organisation going by the acronym of OPEC (Organization of the Petroleum Exporting Countries).

The impact of such a sudden development affected innumerable corners of activity and one of them was the London medical practice.

The emirates, treasuries suddenly overflowing with money, had in one way or another to pass on some of the benefit to their populations where the most immediate demand was for health care. The demand was pressing, the funds available, and it was not possible to wait for the building of new hospitals and the training of doctors. Disease cannot be put on hold so patients were sent in huge numbers to London which had the capacity to handle the influx and where they felt particularly comfortable.

Arab dress tends to be egalitarian in nature so that the arrival in London of relatively large numbers of both men and women led many to assume they were all millionaire "sheikhs" whereas the true situation was quite different. The vast majority were retainers of the sheikhs and emirs for whom health care of this calibre was a windfall. Among them was a group of deaf children and young adults who had never had medical attention, amplification or teaching of any kind so they were all mute, relying on a very primitive form of spontaneous hand signals to communicate.

Hearing aids had been widely available in England for more than 20 years by then, and all but the most profoundly deaf children had received sophisticated teaching with the help of powerful amplification from a very young age.

The new arrivals, on the contrary, had never heard a word and while some were very young and we could place them in the same type of programme of tuition and hearing that we ran in this country with teachers and therapists who spoke Arabic, many were much older.

This gave us a unique opportunity to see how well they did in relation to their ages. Taking into account severity of hearing loss and differences in intelligence, the results were quite striking and we found that the younger they were, the better they did. After the age of seven or eight the chances of learning to speak were very poor.

That was indeed a unique experience, and in England today success in speaking depends more on the severity of the hearing loss, the intelligence of the child, the support of the family and the quality of the teaching than on the age.

5.5 A Language Instinct

In our own time Noam Chomsky made an exceptional contribution to the understanding of language development.

He pointed out that as each sentence is formed as a new combination of words, we must be born with a programme already in our brains causing us to place words in such a meaningful manner. This programme allows us to produce an unlimited number of sentences, all meaningful, even though we have only a finite number of words which we have learnt to put together to make these sentences. It may be thought of as a mental grammar and as all languages are based on this structure it must be common to all humans.

Now that attempts are being made to look for other forms of intelligent life in the universe the problem of communication may arise. If our languages are all based on a common mental programme and if extraterrestrials do not have it we will not be able to translate it as we do foreign languages.

According to the theory of an inborn mental programme leading to a universal grammar, children should develop language in all its complexity quickly and without formal instruction, providing there are consistent patterns in the way the sentences are put together. If we look at the way children speak we can see how these patterns are demonstrated.

Furthermore all languages are complex and the idea of a language evolving from a Stone Age simplicity is made very unlikely by the extreme complexity of those spoken by otherwise very primitive people.

Steven Pinker, who studies the development of language in children, believes there is a language instinct. This would allow each newly born to re-invent language instinctively generation after generation.

He describes many experiments designed to study the responses of newly born babies to speech sounds. These studies have been carried out using rubber nipples connected to recorders which make a mark every time the baby sucks.

Repetitive sounds such as *ba ba ba ba* are played to tiny babies and as they get bored they suck more slowly. If the syllables are changed, even to something very similar such as *pa pa pa pa* they wake up and suck more vigorously.

The *pa* and the *ba* produced by English voices are often not recognisable by other linguistic cultures. The French *papa* is quite different in English where it sounds more like *p-ha p-ha* and yet small babies below six months can recognise the difference.

Pinker also refers to work done by French psychologists demonstrating that even four-day old French babies will show more interest and suck harder if they hear French voices than Russian ones. Presumably the melodies of their French mothers' voices have been carrying through into the womb and the baby is truly born French-speaking! Interestingly, non-French babies have also been shown to prefer their own language but if the words of their own language are played backwards they do not respond in the same way as they do when they sound normal.

Cultural effects get stronger with time and Japanese babies who are able to distinguish between *l* and *r* lose that skill as the months go by, joining the rest of the Japanese population who confuse the two consonants.

Babies begin to understand words before their first birthday and even start to pronounce them. This stage varies widely in time and can last from a few months to a year. Between the ages of 18 months and two years the vocabulary increases very rapidly adding new words every few hours provided, of course, that they can hear them and that they are being spoken around them. Soon the babies begin to put two words together into little sentences, but there is evidence that they can understand them even before they utter them. By the age of three the child should be speaking.

Although a baby may be born with a brain structure which includes that of an innate language, it requires maturation before it can function. Otherwise a baby would be born speaking instead of not even being able to babble. Furthermore, a deaf baby would also speak if its brain at birth were already fully formed.

All nerve cells are already there at birth and they have placed themselves in the right positions in the brain, but the junctions between them, the synapses, are not yet fully developed. These are of crucial importance as it is through these innumerable connections and the networks that result that the brain's computing power is established. Their growth continues and indeed is enhanced after birth at least until the age of two when there is some gradual decrease as the two year old has many more synapses than the adult.

The nerve fibres themselves, prolongations of the nerve cells, may have to travel considerable distances to synapse with the next cell, but as the nerve impulse is an electrical one, the fibres need to be insulated from each other to prevent short circuits just as in any electrical wiring system. This insulation is given by a sheath of a fatty substance called myelin like the rubber sheaths that protect copper wires in our household appliances. Until the whole system is insulated with myelin it is not working adequately. This myelinating process continues throughout childhood.

During the last century, war and the fragmentation of large colonial empires led to the displacement of people on an unprecedented scale; indeed I myself am one of them. The displacement gave me an opportunity to observe at close quarters how people of different ages responded to new languages. Those of school age and even those already in their 20s were able to master the vocabulary and grammar of their new countries with hardly any difficulty. However, they rarely achieved impeccable accents if they had arrived after puberty.

Even successful writers who have made major contributions to the literature of their new country retained thick foreign accents — Joseph Conrad and Vladimir Nabokov are two such examples.

This indicates that quite a high level of maturation takes place during the establishment of the learnt language or languages onto the basic universal structure of the brain networks during a period of plasticity. After the period of maturation has ended it is of course quite possible to learn new languages but the sounds and phonological aspects appear to be fixed.

The importance of appreciating this developmental process has been greatest in our understanding of the mechanism of language deprivation and particularly in our management and education of the deaf child.

5.6 Bilingualism and Prejudice

I was once asked to teach a course on child development for community physicians where I was to discuss the assessment of children who has failed to develop speech.

The organiser had written to me explaining that I was required to talk about deafness, but I was intrigued by her insistence that I need not concern myself with other possible causes such as global mental disability, autism and language deprivation which would be dealt with by others. There was an array of better qualified experts, she implied, to deal with these matters and all they wanted from me was how to check whether children could hear or not.

I did what she had asked although it was difficult to avoid other aspects entirely as we approach the child as a whole rather than as separate systems, and I mentioned that quite a few children with a hearing loss had initially been missed because they had been diagnosed as "bilingual" as though it was a disease. All I had wanted to say was that if a child's speech was delayed it should be investigated as it could be deaf, for instance, or it may suffer by other developmental problems; it should not dismissed simply because the parents spoke another language at home.

Most of the doctors in my audience came from the Indian sub-continent or other countries and they were particularly interested in bilingualism so at question time, that was their main concern.

I explained that exposure to more than one language was not harmful in itself. A large section of the world population was brought up in the presence of different languages with no ill effects and I gave myself as an example.

After they filed out of the lecture hall the organiser had stayed behind.

"I waited because I did not want to embarrass you," she said, "but your English accent is not absolutely perfect. What I want to ask is whether your French is?"

I confessed that I hoped it was imperceptible but I doubted it was perfect in French either.

"I thought so!" she said, and stumped out triumphantly.

5.7 Broca's Brain

Not long ago the French newspapers reported that Dr Paul Broca's brain had been found in a jar.

The formalin in which it had been pickled was leaking, and according to the paper the brain was rescued just as it was about to be thrown away.

The press tends to dramatise events, turning an obscure story into an interesting, if ephemeral feature, and this brain was not Dr Broca's own brain but that of one of his patients, which appeared to have been misplaced for more than 100 years.

It was the examination of this brain that led to an important part of modern neurology. The man whose organ it was had lost the capacity for speech and the only syllable he uttered while in hospital was "tan". His condition is referred to as "aphasia".

When the patient died, Dr Broca examined the brain and found that part of the left side, known as the left hemisphere, had been destroyed by a cyst. When he had the opportunity of dissecting the brains of other aphasic patients he found that they all had lesions in the left hemisphere. It was 140 years ago that Broca had noted this association and concluded that "the faculty for articulate language" was found in the left hemisphere of the brain. The area responsible for speech has since been known as Broca's area.

We now know that this faculty for speech also applies to deaf patients who cannot speak and rely on signing. A lesion affecting the left hemisphere will impair their sign language even though the motor skills of their hand may not be weakened otherwise.

The right hemisphere is responsible for visuo-spatial skills and if damaged both those who can hear and those who are deaf will be affected in the same way.

This means that the left hemisphere controls language in its most basic form and the rules which decide grammar as well as our vocabulary reside there. Today neuroscientists consider aphasia as more complex than just Broca's area and involves more deep seated pathways and connections. There are also subtle differences in the aphasia which results when a number of other areas of the brain are damaged.

5.8 The Voice

Sometimes people, especially children, are said not to be "speaking properly" when it is the voice that is the problem.

The normal voice should have a pleasing quality and not be harsh or hoarse or breathy. It should achieve the level of loudness required of it, and its pitch should be appropriate for age, size and sex. It should also have the proper inflections and prosody.

The voice is produced by the larynx, a cartilage tube of a rather complex shape which gradually becomes ossified. Colloquially but not unreasonably, the larynx is often referred to as the "voice box". The front end of it which sticks out is called the Adam's apple as it is more prominent in men.

The larynx leads downwards to the chest through another tube-like cartilaginous passage, the trachea, and this in turn divides into two bronchi that end up in the lungs (Figure 20).

When we breathe in and out air passes from our nose and mouth through the larynx, trachea and bronchi to the lungs and then blows out again the same way.

This movement of air is brought about by the muscles of respiration. There are many, large and small, as even some of the neck muscles help in pulling up the chest, but better known are the diaphragm which also

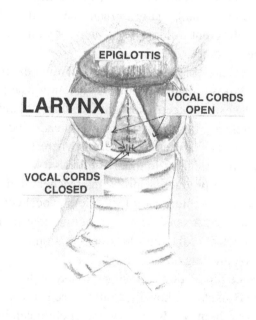

Figure 20 Larynx.

separates the cavity of the chest from that of the abdomen and the muscles between the ribs which expand and contract the chest wall, sucking the air in and squeezing it out. What makes them do this, either on purpose or subconsciously, is the brain but as they all have to work together in a coordinated manner rather than fight each other, they are controlled by the same parts of the brain which can be called the respiratory centres.

This applies to all animals but in humans there was a special development of the tiny uppermost respiratory muscles which pull the larynx open to breathe or close it to prevent unwanted particles from slipping down into the lungs.

Two muscles in particular can come together in the middle, closing off the larynx altogether at will. When we breathe in or out we pull them apart so that the air can pass through unhindered. If we keep them together, forcing the air past them, we make a sound. This is the voice and we call these two muscles the vocal cords.

During the course of evolution from primitive animals to ape-like creatures, various hominids and finally to man, the vocal cords have become able to produce different volumes of sound as well as, by tensing and relaxing, different pitches.

Even though we are able to control and fine-tune the movement of the vocal cords, our voice sometimes indicates emotion whether we want it to or not. It is much easier to keep a straight face than a bland voice if we are anxious or frightened. Those who are naturally endowed and well trained are able to control their voices to an extent where their singing abilities can induce powerful emotions in their listeners.

In rectifying voice production problems teachers and voice therapists often rely on the basic evolutionary fact that the vocal cords were initially muscles of respiration. A sensible way of getting a grip on the voice is to try to get better control of the muscles of respiration as a whole since they share the same controlling areas in the brain.

Abnormal voice production can be due to psychological causes, which is not surprising considering how much the voice is involved in expressing emotion with or without words. A very young child can burst into tears at its mother's angry voice even if it does not understand a word she is saying and it will be soothed into comfort and sleep by loving words and a lullaby.

Voice changes can also result from physical lesions such as swelling or thickening of the vocal cords resulting from infection or allergy or even too much shouting. Nodules or polyps or even cancers can occur on the vocal cords and they can sometimes suffer paralysis. All of these can be recognised by a specialist as the larynx is easily seen with the new fibre optic endoscopes and often with a simple mirror.

5.9 Speech

If language can be considered the defining tool developed as a means of communication then speech is the most successful way of using language.

The relationship between language and speech is uniquely human. This has led to considerable questioning as to which primates or hominids in the evolutionary scale had the mechanism permitting them to speak and were therefore "human".

Efforts have been made to teach language to gorillas and chimpanzees but this may miss the point. Of course animals can learn many things and have remarkable memories, just as they show other human traits such as having strong emotions such as affection.

Some animals can relate and communicate with us better than others, hence our close relationships with the dog and the horse rather than with tigers and leopards. That does not mean that dogs and horses have the language structures in the brain that humans have. These animals cannot develop language and the fact that the dog does not have an appropriate mouth either and therefore cannot utter words is irrelevant to its lack of human language.

Every time a new hominid skeleton is discovered, a discussion starts as to whether it had language or not, as if it did it could be defined as human. The question of whether its anatomical structures would allow it to speak like us is not important as there can be no speech if there is no inner language. On the other hand it would really not matter if its mouth and throat were not able to voice words as the existence of such an inner language, no matter how it were expressed, is what defines humanity. The evidence we should be looking for is the individual's capacity to create symbols such as pictures on a cave wall or to decide the shape of a stone axe and go on to create it, rather than merely basing supposition on jaw measurements.

Language, of course, can exist perfectly well in the absence of speech as in the case of the profoundly deaf where they are able to express themselves by gesture. Indeed, even when speech is present, gesture can contribute a great deal in the enhancement of meaning or feeling and some societies use hand movements, shrugging of shoulders and so on more than others.

I suspect that an Italian deaf person might find it easier to follow what his countrymen mean than his English equivalent as much more can be gleaned from the gestures made by Mediterranean people when they speak compared to their northern European counterparts.

I attended a lecture by a distinguished French scientist who lived and worked in the south of the country when I saw him looking troubled as he tried to direct a pointer to a slide he had projected. He finally gave up his effort, put down the pointer, shrugged his shoulders and explained the difficult concept he was discussing with obvious relief and a profusion of gestures.

"Not to be able to use the hands in speech is a problem for someone from the south!" he explained.

He told me that until that moment he had not realised that the movement of his hands actually helped him to formulate the words and sentences transforming inner language into speech.

Producing speech itself involves the use of many structures: the voice, the mouth and the throat.

5.9.1 *The sounds of speech*

The production of speech sounds starts with the movement of air. This can be achieved with the mouth alone or by the air we push out of the lungs and past the closed or open vocal cords. In English all the speech sounds are produced in this way, and, indeed most sounds in other languages too. There are altogether 30 or so such sounds.

We can modify the sound by altering the tautness of the vocal cords so as to change the pitch and this itself imparts some information. For instance raising the tone at the end of a sentence suggests a question rather than a statement.

All the sounds of speech, in all languages, are grouped into two major classes, the consonants and the vowels.

The consonants are produced by restriction or closure of the air passages whereas when we make vowel sounds the flow remains unrestricted even while we change the shape of the vocal tract in order to obtain different sounds.

5.9.1.1 *Consonant sounds*

We can alter the sound of the voice by movements of the lips, tongue and palate, changing the shape and volume of the cavity of the mouth.

In this way, to make the sound *p* and *b* as well as *m,* we bring the lips together as the air pushing past the vibrating vocal cords reaches the mouth. To make the sounds *v* and *f* we place our bottom lip against our upper teeth. If we want to make the sounds *t, d, n, l* and *r* we raise the front of the tongue towards the back of the teeth.

These sounds are all consonants and we make them by changing the shape of the mouth by moving the lips and tongue. The sounds are changed by the position of the tongue and soft palate. We can even change sounds without using the voice at all. For instance by bringing the lips together the sound that comes out is *b* but if we make the same mouth movements, this time avoiding producing a voice by keeping the vocal cord open, and just spitting out the air, what emerges is a *p.*

To make an *m* we bring the lips together just as in *b* and we also make a voice at the same time and yet these two consonants do not sound the same. This is because in *m* we let the air escape through our nose as we speak whereas when we want to say *b* we raise our soft palate to close off the nasal airway. The same effect happens when we have a cold so that when we try to say "*man*" it comes out *ban.*

If the soft palate is inadequate, for instance if it has not developed properly so that a child is born with a cleft or is malformed in other ways so that it cannot close off the nose during speech, the opposite will happen. It is called "nasal escape" and this time "ban" will sound like "man".

From time to time surgeons fail to realise that there are two types of nasal speech and we come across a problem. Most cases of "nasal" speech in children occur when the nose is blocked by enlarged adenoids. Strictly speaking it should be called "hypo-nasal" as there is too little air passing through the nose. The proper treatment is to remove the adenoids and this is often done as the condition is so common.

Sadly, occasionally we find that a rather hasty surgeon has not realised that the problem was "hyper" and not "hypo-nasal" speech. In other words, the palate's movement was inadequate and the abnormal sounding consonants are not the result of blockage but rather of too much air escape. Intemperate excision of the adenoids will make matters worse, not better.

This aspect of speech is referred to as "articulation" and the consonant sounds are divided into classes. For instance the *p*, *b* and *m* sounds are called "bilabials" because we use both lips to make them, while the *f* and *v* are called "labiodentals". The other classes are the "interdentals", "alveolar", "palatal", and "velar" according to the lip, tongue and soft palate position.

Other languages also have "uvular" sounds made at the back of the throat. In French, the Parisians make their *r* in that way, and Arabic, which has two *r*'s, makes one of them similarly. Arabic has two *k*'s as well and again one of them is a uvular.

The *h* sound as in "hair" or "who" allows the air to pass straight through the gap between the vocal cords, which is also known as the glottis and so it is called "glottal". The cockney East End of London speech evolved in its own peculiar manner and words like "button" are pronounced "bu'on". The gap were the *tt* should have been is achieved by closing the vocal cords tightly so that no sound at all comes out. This is known as a "glottal stop".

Thus consonant sounds are differentiated both by the position of mouth and lips and also by the way the air stream is handled; in other words, the voice.

If the vocal cords are apart and the glottis not obstructed the sounds are called "voiceless" and they include *p*, *t*, *k* and *s*.

If the cords are closed they vibrate when air is forced past them and the sounds made by the same lip movements become *b*, *d*, *g* and *z*. These, then, with the added vibration of the cords are called "voiced" sounds.

The difference between voiced and voiceless sounds is very important to the deaf lip-reader. He can tell that the lips are making the sound *s* or *z* but not which one so that the girl's name "Sue" and the word "zoo" look the same and can lead to confusion. When we started developing the cochlear implant some critics felt that our work was not worth the effort as the amount of hearing we could offer then was still minimal. On the other hand we could show that it was useful even if all that was available was the difference between voiced and voiceless sounds.

By making the air pass through a very narrow passage in the mouth it can cause turbulent friction so that sounds like *f*, *v*, *s*, *z* and *th* are also referred to as "fricatives".

The *l* and the *r* are called "liquids" and cause considerable confusion to Japanese and Cantonese speakers as they have only one liquid consonant and they become unable to distinguish between our two.

Some English speakers can have problems pronouncing the *r* which comes out as a *w*. There has also been a shift in certain parts of London as when the *l* is the terminal sound in a word such as "a mea*l*" or "St Paul's Cathedral" it changes to a *w* and becomes "a mea*ow*" and "St Pau*w*'s Cathedral". The *w* is known as a "glide" or a "semivowel" because it is always preceded or followed by a vowel.

There are consonant sounds that we do not use in speech. The sound "sk" as in "tsk, tsk, tsk" is an example. It is never used as part of a word but it represents a clear cut expression in itself and it is definitely negative. During my childhood in Egypt I quickly discovered that the expression "tsk!" uttered with a very slight toss of the head simply meant "no!" It was widely used in the streets but strongly discouraged at home.

In some South African languages, such as Xhosa and Khoikhoi, clicks are used as parts of words and true consonants. Indeed, the name Xhosa itself starts with one.

5.9.1.2 *Vowels*

The passage of air is never obstructed when we make vowel sounds even though we change the shape of our mouths and lips in order to make them. We can open our lips or purse them and we can raise or lower different parts of the tongue. As they are made by the voice we can sing them and we can make them long as in "s*ea*t" or short as in "s*i*t". Because of the role that the position of the tongue has they are often referred to as "high" and "low" or "front" and "back".

When I ask a patient to say "ah" it makes him lower the tongue so it is easier for me to see the back so we call "ah" a low, back vowel. On the other hand if I need to look down at his vocal cords with a laryngeal mirror I have to pull his tongue forward above his lower teeth and if he says "ah" he pulls it back in. That is why we ask the patient to "ee" instead. This raises the front part of the tongue so that "ee" is a high front vowel.

If we say the back vowel "ah" but at the same time we purse or round our lips we get different sounds. These are called "rounded vowels" and we get the "oo", "uh", "er" and so on.

It is with trepidation that I write these vowels down as professionals give them special written forms. I am also likely to confuse and irritate some people as we all have our own dialects and accents. George Bernard Shaw expressed the problem in his play *Pygmalion* where he has Pickering saying to Professor Higgins, "I rather fancied myself because I can pronounce twenty-four distinct vowel sounds, but your hundred and thirty beat me. I can't hear a bit of difference between them." Higgins tells him that if you keep listening you will eventually be able to do so. In the film musical *My Fair Lady*, which was adapted from the play, Audrey Hepburn gave a remarkable rendering of a considerable number of vowel sounds heard in London.

This leads us to the problem we have with trying to express all the varied pronunciations that exist even in our own language when we write. Again, Shaw thought he had a solution. He showed his contempt for our alphabet in the preface he wrote for *Pygmalion*:

> "The English have no respect for their language, and will not teach their children to speak it. They cannot spell it because they have nothing to spell it with but an old foreign alphabet of which only the consonants — and not all of them — have any agreed speech value."

He left some money in his will for a new alphabet which he thought should have at least 40 letters to cover all the speech sounds but nothing came of it.

In fact the International Phonetics Association (IPA) had prepared such an alphabet at the end of the 19th century, which was subsequently revised in 1989. The symbols are useful to professionals but cannot be used in the general world. After all, the written word has a meaning of its own separate from the exact sound which can be varied by different people. It should be written the same to be read by all English speakers, by speakers of other languages and by the deaf, however they may sound.

5.9.2 Learning to speak

The number of words we know is finite, although we can always learn more words, provided we have the capacity to remember them all. Words are stored in our brain as a sort of dictionary and acquiring new words is a straightforward business.

This does not apply to sentences. Every sentence we hear is a new thought expressed by someone, which we are able to understand and have not heard before. The words we have all learnt must be put in a certain order and follow certain rules, and it is this set of rules that we call grammar.

How this grammar was learnt remained an awesome mystery until the 1950s and 1960s when the theory of an inborn system based on the structure of the brain, common to all humans and not to other animals, answered many questions. For example a child will have learnt that to add -*ed* to the end of a verb places it in the past. It will do this correctly when it says "I walk*ed*" or "I jump*ed*" and if it learns a new verb it will add -*ed* in the same way when it wants to indicate the past because of its acceptance of the system of grammatical rules. So much so that it will make "mistakes" in following the rules correctly by saying "I runn*ed*" and "I leav*ed*". These very errors suggest that the child is trying to construct sentences according to grammatical rules.

Learning words and putting them into grammatical sentences rather than gibberish is a very distinct process that follows definite stages even though they may overlap.

5.9.2.1 Babbling

It seems that babies can distinguish between human voices and other sounds virtually from birth as the experiments with sucking on rubber nipples have shown. Very soon their articulatory system allows them to imitate speech sounds and by the age of six months they have started to reproduce them as babbling.

We know that making these sounds is a response to hearing them as we have observed that deaf babies do not make the sounds. We also know that they have to practise making them, as children who have had to have a tracheostomy can be delayed in speech production. A tracheostomy means inserting a breathing tube into the trachea and therefore these children cannot speak until the tube can be taken out or blocked in a temporary manner.

Different languages include different sounds but some are more common to all. Vowels are more difficult to assess as they are similar to spontaneous cooing and whimpering, but the most common consonants are: *p*, *b*, *m*, *t*, *d*, *n*, *k*, *g* and also *s*, *h*, *w*, *j*. It is therefore not surprising to find them in babble of all nations. On the other hand some consonants like *f*, *v*, *th*, *l* and *r* are much rarer and yet appear in the early babble, just as Japanese babies are able to recognise and produce both *l* and *r*, a skill which they subsequently lose.

5.9.2.2 *Words*

Babbling becomes more frequent as the months pass and by the age of one year we can perceive understandable words.

Acquisition of words is now extremely rapid and by the time the baby has around 50 repeatable words the babbling fades away and gradually disappears. Pronunciation now follows regular patterns.

Vowels seem to appear before consonants and by the age of two, English speaking children are able to articulate *p*, *b*, *m*, *t*, *d*, *n*, *k*, *g*, *f*, *s* and *w*. By the age of four they have added other sounds including *l*, *r* and *j*.

Small children find some segments of speech more difficult to articulate than others and so they simplify them. "Stop" becomes "top", "from" becomes "fom", "sleep" becomes "seep" and so on. They just delete the difficult syllable but it is usually the final consonant that is deleted. "Dog" becomes "do'" and "bus" is "bu'". Often the child will substitute a difficult one for an easy one. A common one is to substitute the *w* for the *r* as in "sto*w*y" instead of "sto*r*y". This may persist for a long time.

5.9.2.3 *One- and two-word stage*

Although the child will start making only one-word utterances between the ages of one year and eighteen months they show an increasing complexity.

Other meaningful sounds are bound to the words. An -*s* is added to make a plural and for the possessive. Eventually the past tense arrives as -*ed,* and -*ing* appears quite early.

The meaning of single words begins to represents the intent behind a whole sentence so that parents will sometimes insist that they are actually making sentences.

"Dada" can obviously mean "my Daddy has just come in". "Up!" clearly says "pick me up", and when the child says "more" in the right context it is saying "I want more cookies!"

In a similar way, children transition between the one-word stage and the two-word stage between eighteen months and two years. They begin to make real small sentences such as "Mummy busy" or "Daddy push".

5.9.2.4 *The telegraphic stage*

After the age of two, the child, who has been learning new words extremely rapidly and adding them to its mental store, will be making sentences of three or more words and they will put them immediately in the right grammatical order for the language. The child will say "Mimi push chair" and never "push chair Mimi" unless it belongs to a language group that places words in that order.

It will not, at first, use words like "a" and "the" and so the speech will sound like "telegraphese", but by two and a half definite and indefinite articles begin to appear and language development is very rapid.

5.9.2.5 *Later development*

The order of words continues to develop and becomes more complex. Questions and statement can be distinguished, and by the age of three we should be able to say that the child can speak.

The development of language does not take place in isolation, and articulation is part of the emergence of other motor skills but most important in this context is the simultaneous course of cognitive development.

Cognitive development is the name given to the appearance of the mental skills and capacity that are the human intellect. As there are equally important changes taking place in the non-linguistic field some psychologists believe that the two are interdependent. Some say that language acquisition is simply a part of general cognitive development while others would reverse the concept by saying that the acquisition of language drives the rest of cognitive development.

Initially children believe that what they cannot see does not exist. This means that they cannot look for a hidden object even though they may have seen it being hidden. At around 18 months a child develops the ability to understand the concept that an object is permanent and that it remains somewhere even though it cannot be seen. Interestingly, it is about that time that the child's vocabulary increases rapidly and it starts naming objects.

By the age of two the child is able to classify objects into groups. It knows what objects are toys, even in other peoples' houses, and what are edible foodstuffs and what are not. At the same the child will classify words into groups and knows the difference between nouns, for instance, and "doing" words (verbs). The child now knows that dogs, cats and other living creatures are all animals even though they each make a different sound and look different. ("What does the dog say? Woof! Woof!") It knows that the teddy bear is not an animal but an inanimate object even though it looks and feels like an animal.

As it puts words together into sentences it is putting bricks together into towers and then bridges and can tell the difference between "big" and "small" or between "long" and "short".

By the age of five the child is able to classify objects in order of bigness or length and is aware of the existence of series and of degrees. At the same time it also begins to understand words such as "longer" or "smaller".

The ability to classify is quite remarkable as I found once when asking a six-year-old whether any of his friends had robot dogs. He had never seen one other than on television but he understood exactly what it was.

His four year old sister seemed confused but as soon as the word "robot" was explained to her she grasped the problem immediately. She had understood that I was not referring to a real dog but to an inanimate object, a toy, that could simulate the movement and behaviour of a real one.

It seemed that my description of what the new word "robot" meant was what led the little girl to understand the whole problem and immediately to classify the toy dog in her mind even though she had never seen one. In her case, words and language had a preeminent role in facilitating if not actually driving her intellectual skills.

I am curious to see at what age children recognise the place robot animals have, once they become a commonplace item. The introduction of new technologies must inevitably affect the way children will develop and, aside from robots that may replace animals, I understand that practice with computer games is greatly improving skills that require eye–finger coordination.

5.10 Gesture

One night I was desperately trying to hail a taxi in Syntagma Square in Athens. I was anxious about my lateness and frustrated by the taxis that did not stop. After a while, I was approached by a man.

"You German?" he asked.
"No," I said.
"You want go to go cabaret?"
"No! No!"
"I get you women," he insisted.
"I don't want women!"
"Never mind," he whispered conspiratorially. "I get you boys."
"I only want a taxi!" I shouted. "Just leave me alone!"

As I spoke I gestured with the palm of my hand towards him, fingers spread out as though to push him away. This infuriated him and he took hold of my coat and I thought he was going to hit me.

"You do '*NA!*' to me as though I am nothing?" He was beginning to rough me up. "I am not nothing, I am owner of cabaret! You not do '*NA!*' to me!"

My gesture must have symbolised disdain rather than dismissal and was more offensive than my intention, but my apologies were not enough when inspiration took me.

"You said I was German, when I am British!"

Suddenly he stopped, pensive, weighing up which offence was the more serious, my disdainful gesture or his mistake.

I apologised again and he fortunately came to the conclusion that I too had been justified in taking offence. He said that it was not always easy to tell the difference as we look the same, and ran towards a taxi that had stopped at the lights and ushered me in.

5.10.1 *Symbolic gestures*

Symbolic gestures of this type show differences between generations as well as cultures, though it could be argued that to some extent generations may count as different cultures.

I was saddened at one man in my clinic at Guy's Hospital as I noticed that the older patients had thanked me as they left, while this shaven-headed young man had not bothered to do so.

"But he did thank you!" the students said in one voice, explaining that the young man's thumbs up gesture represented gratitude together with the muttered words:

"Cheers, mate!"

I have learnt to respond by raising my own thumb and sometimes I also say "Cheers!"

It is a question of learning the language of gestures, although many of the gestures can be quite rude.

Winston Churchill popularised the V-sign during the war to such an extent that it acquired an enormous emotional content. The power of those two raised fingers throughout the world was so great that the Nazi propagandists tried to appropriate it by introducing the word *Victoria* when the German word for victory is *zieg*. It did not work. Perhaps it lacked the other distinctive symbols of the cigar and, of course, the man himself.

A boy at my junior school told me that there was a deeper, secret meaning to two raised fingers that is considered quite rude, and the grownups knew what he really meant. Unfortunately his information was limited, and he was unable to tell me what Churchill was secretly indicating. It was many years before I discovered the sexual innuendo of a two-finger gesture.

In recent years it is a single finger, usually the middle finger, which is raised in an insulting manner. I have wondered why the middle finger seems so much more offensive than the index finger which is easier to raise. Perhaps the index finger is commonly used in pointing so the middle finger is more emphatic.

These gestures, however silly, will drive otherwise reasonable men to fury and many instances of road rage have been initiated by the unexpected emotional power of such gestural symbolism.

Of course, there are other, more agreeable signals and gestures used in everyday life, such as the raised hand to thank a driver who has allowed us into the flow of traffic, or the slight inclination of the trunk with movement of the hand when we invite someone to precede us through a door.

We show affection or consolation by hugging. Kisses on the cheek between men and women are now a recognised sign of even slight acquaintance in England. This "kissing the air", or "Muah! Muah!" as it is sometimes referred to, has also come to indicate an element of hypocrisy since it has become so meaningless.

I am told that the degree of incline in the Japanese bow indicates relative status, which is recognised by both parties.

In the West the handshake indicates some degree of trust and, although it is a democratic gesture which probably originated in Britain as an affirmation such as the "let us shake on it" of a contract, it is now widely used everywhere.

Yet touching between men and women is not universally acceptable and I was asked to deal with a crisis when I arrived at the operating theatre one morning. An Iranian visiting surgeon explained that he was not prepared to shake hands with the scrub nurse to whom he was to be introduced as his religious scruples did not allow him to touch women but he was anxious not to cause offence. We agreed that an inclination of the head and a friendly smile was sufficient.

Such reticent nodding is acceptable in Britain but might seem disdainful to the French who shake hands a great deal more. My brother, who went to school in Paris, told me that even the little boys in the junior school would go round the class every morning, shaking hands with each one in turn.

When I was a medical student we never shook hands with the patients as it was considered to be intrusive. We could examine their private parts but shaking hands was too intimate.

One consultant who had a very large private practice told us confidentially that the secret of his success was that he shook hands twice with each one of his patients. As they came in and when they left.

"It draws them close to you," he had said. "Like a fond relative!"

"Smarmy bastard!" I heard students mutter.

Today, medical students are shown videos that insist shaking the hand of the patient is absolutely essential.

We do not bow or curtsey any longer but it was the rule in the 18th century, as evidenced by mentions of such manners in Jane Austen's books. I once had to introduce some of my child patients to a member of royalty. All the mothers curtseyed although they had not been asked to do so. They did it impeccably so they must have practised and the royal lady took it in her stride, indicating that she was used to this sort of behaviour.

The formal bowing and curtseying of the 18th and early 19th centuries was itself an innovation. Indeed the Byzantine historian and writer Procopius had accompanied the Emperor Manuel as he travelled round Christendom to raise money for the defence of Constantinople. He noted that in medieval England women, whether high born or low, were inclined to embrace visitors and kiss them on both cheeks. He insisted that the foreigner should not be misled into thinking that it represented flirtatiousness. Now we can see that the practice has come full circle: hugging and kissing visitors on the cheeks has returned to our culture.

5.10.2 *Enhancing speech*

Aside from gestures as symbols (i.e. as visual signs that represent concepts of their own) we use gesture to enhance what we are saying. A fist banging on a table is an obvious example or, even more striking, Khrushchev banging his desk with his shoe at the United Nations Assembly in 1960. There are countless hand gestures that we use automatically as we speak, like the index finger wagged at a naughty child but other parts of the body also take part, such as frowning and shrugging.

Interestingly, the English, at least since the 19th century, taught that there was something vulgar or excessive about gesture as part of speech, associated no doubt with the culture of a stiff upper lip. Few other languages showed such inhibitions.

With the introduction of brain scans of different types there has been a revival of interest in the role of gesture as enhancing or broadening meaning and the question arises as to whether it is helpful to the speaker or the listener or indeed both. This is not as esoteric as it may seem as it will help us understand and treat stroke victims and perhaps patients who fall on the autistic spectrum.

5.10.3 *The beginning of language*

In 1866 the *Societé Linguistique de Paris* simply banned debates on the origins of language because there was no evidence on which to base any reasonable discussion.

An unusual thing to do, it is an example everyone should forever keep in mind, though it could not stop the lunatic fringe developing its own theories and in the early 1900s Jean-Pierre Brisset came to an extraordinary conclusion.

He had been sitting in the countryside when a frog looked him straight in the eye and said "*coac*". There was nothing surprising about that, of course, as Brisset knew that it was what frogs said but as he listened more attentively and when the animal repeated "*coac-coac*" he realised that the frog was actually saying "*quoi?*" or "what?" and then became convinced that "*coac-coac-coac*" was in fact "*quoi que tu dis?*" or "what are you saying?"

That encounter led Brisset, an eclectic pastry-chef and inventor, to take an interest in linguistics and he eventually concluded that humanity was more likely descended from frogs than from apes and he proved to his own satisfaction that the French language, at least, originated entirely from the "*coac-coac*" of frogs.

In 1913 a group of sophisticated highbrows decided to make fun of him. Electing him "*Prince of Philosophers*" they invited him to a dinner where they all mocked him in flowery speeches all of which, together with his ingenuous response, were published in a satirical magazine the following day. This true story resembles Verber's film *le Dîner de Cons,* which the Americans remade as *The Dinner Game.* The American version was less successful, as no one can be as merciless and unkind towards the less urbane or uneducated than a Parisian elite.

Nevertheless, we still wonder how language began, though we have more facts at our disposal than in 1866. We have hopes of being able to do something about speech and language problems if we understood them better. The fundamental debate remains the same one for evolutionists: did language evolve gradually from primitive grunts to the complexities of modern languages or was there a sudden genetic mutation when *Homo sapiens* emerged, somewhere between 100,000 and 200,000 years ago, that gave our mutant ancestor such a powerful new tool allowing him or her to finally break away from and eventually dominate the rest of the animal kingdom.

Statistical computer analysis suggests that languages began to diversify about 100,000 years ago corresponding with genetic and paleontological evidence of the emergence of mankind. It has also confirmed that there are no primitive languages as every single one, whether ancient or modern, is equally complex and has the same expressive powers.

Some believe that a language of gesture may have come first, as certain postures, like that of begging, appear to be the same everywhere and must be closer to an original mother tongue for all humanity.

It came as a surprise to me that most of the evidence points to a sudden mutation that granted us language in one go, though when we consider how much evolution depends on random mutation it is not so unbelievable. The strongest evidence for this conclusion is that which comes from recent genetic findings.

5.10.3.1 *FOXP2*

FOXP2 is found on the autosomal chromosome 7 in a section called SPCH1 and can be identified in all mammals. It regulates many target genes including one called CNTNAP2, which has been associated with common forms of language impairment and is expressed in many parts of the brain. That gene is also connected to a large extended family which is called KE or just K where over three generations half the members have suffered speech and language deficits in what appeared to be autosomal dominant transmission. In the early 1990s Oxford geneticists Simon Fisher and Anthony Monaco and their colleagues described the connection with FOXP2 and language production. The Mendelian inheritance of a mutation where damage to one copy of the gene is enough to disturb both speech and language development.

Those members of the KE family with no abnormality had inherited a normal gene while those with the mutation all suffered muscular weakness around the mouth causing verbal dyspraxia as well as difficulty in comprehension while MRI scans showed functional abnormalities in the language related areas of the brain.

These discoveries not only help us to understand the causes of disability and bring us a step nearer to treating them, but also point to the origin of language, as the two are clearly intertwined.

Genetics has advanced so far that we now know that although chimpanzees and other animals share FOXP2 with us they do not have the mutation that has given us language. On the other hand Neanderthal man and their contemporaries, the Denisovan hominids of the Far East, could have, and indeed did, interbreed with *Homo sapiens* of which they must have been a fellow sub-species.

It is likely, then, that language, which transformed animals into humans, came as a mutation, a gift bestowed all of a sudden to our species perhaps 200,000 years ago.

Chapter 6

Music and the Sound of Feelings

Music is an extraordinary form of communication which uses sound and seems to bypass intellectual analysis, directly evoking emotions. It involves human attributes such as art and culture. Few things have been so widely studied but despite that, the exact mechanism, the way sound vibrations are transformed into feeling, is far from fully understood.

6.1 Music and Birdsong

There is a particular cricket that has a very narrow range of hearing, around 6 kHz to be precise, a very high pitch hardly audible to many people over 60. These crickets can also produce a zizzing sound of the same pitch by rubbing their legs together. They use it as a sexual attractant. That limited range of auditory capacity and sound production is all that the cricket needs to inform possible partners of his presence and invite them to approach him so that they can reproduce.

There is a tiny fly, too, that can focus on the pitch that certain crickets are producing for their own purposes in order to find them and lay their eggs on them.

The innumerable known and as yet unknown uses that animals make of sound are quite different from the role of music in human culture despite occasional romantic beliefs which suggest the contrary.

The most important of these is birdsong. This has always impressed mankind and people have tried to imitate it and been inspired to write their own music on the basis of its melody. Mozart claimed to have incorporated the starling's song in the last movement of his Concerto in G, while

Vivaldi, Bach and Beethoven and countless others have also turned bird-song into music.

Although we are certainly not dealing with the same phenomenon when we compare music with birdsong it is difficult to know where the boundary lies between the conscious communication of emotion from one individual to many, and the narrow, specific instinct which birdsong represents.

Darwin had observed that the vocalisation of chicks, what is called subsong, resembles babbling. By eight months canaries sing adult songs during the breeding and moulting seasons of spring and summer, though only the male sings. He can cover a wide octave range but if females are injected with the male hormone testosterone, a particular part deep inside the brain will grow in size and they will sing too.

The purpose of birdsong is to do with sex and territory and they are very closely related. The song will attract the female in the breeding period and it will also act as a warning to other males to keep away from that couple's territory which will have to produce enough food for the hatchlings.

Many studies have been carried out on the nature of birdsong and have produced very interesting information such as the fact that the male birds get accustomed to their neighbours' songs but if a stranger's sound is introduced it will create an immediate rise in the volume of singing by all the surrounding familiar males. Birdsong is adaptable — according to some newspaper reports a number of starlings in Trafalgar Square have learnt the tunes produced by mobile telephones.

How this works is still unknown. Where does the canary learn a new song each year? Who do they imitate?

6.2 Music as a Human Attribute

Awareness of our environment obviously begins with the ability to perceive things. Touch provides a direct and immediate experience of an object as does sight. Hearing, taste and smell in turn give us information about the qualities of the object.

An appreciation of art is a complex, entirely human phenomenon of which perception is only the first step. When we see a sculpture, for instance, or a painting, we look at it in the context of our own basic values and this leads to an emotional response which may be pleasure, hostility, anger, puzzlement or whatever.

Our response to music is not the same as perception turns directly into emotion which may then be followed by intellectual analysis or not. A piece of music evokes a feeling, an emotion, which is then subconsciously compared with other situations which cause us to experience the same feeling. Beethoven's Sixth Symphony is known as the "Pastoral" because it evokes the same feelings in many people who are familiar with an idyllic countryside. This does not mean that it mimics the bleating of sheep or the mooing of cows or even the sound of running streams. Some people may say that the Sixth Symphony does not produce pastoral feelings in them at all. A great deal depends on the mood of the listener; in any case the stress is on the idyllic and not on the reality of the countryside.

Many surgeons like to have music played in their operating theatres during prolonged surgery but naturally the choice of music varies. I myself liked to have chamber works by Fauré or Saint Saens but I do not know why. Sometimes I have asked for baroque music and occasionally I have requested a very romantic movement by Tchaikovsky. I have not been able to correlate my desire with a particular type of operation so I imagine it is likely to be related to my mood. I think that what I sought while I was operating was likely to be a complex mixture of emotions. I suspect that I needed to be calm rather than anxious but that I also needed to be alert. Clearly I had to feel "good" but in giving this list of requirements I was probably unaware of my most important needs.

The cardiac surgeon who performed brilliantly in the adjoining operating theatre liked to have loud pop music played, often joining in the vocal parts with his assistants as they knew the words well. I found the sound unsettling while I was working and had the heavy doors shut. When I became curious about the need for music I listened more carefully and watched them. I found that they seemed to be carried as on a high, singing as a team but when they came to an especially intricate part of the surgery they would turn the music off completely.

Some perfectly good pieces may appear flippant in certain situations and irritating in others but if they correspond to the emotion within us the effect can be very powerful. We still do not know why music makes us experience emotions in so direct and immediate a manner without the intervention of the intellect or how a particular sequence of sounds can generate in us such sad, joyful or inspiring feelings.

Hermann von Helmholtz, a physicist who lived in the 19th century, believed that the essence of musical perception is mathematical, that the consonance or dissonance which we perceive in harmonies depends on the ratio of the frequencies of their tones. The brain for instance can cope with a ratio of 1:2 but not of 8:9.

The brain has to be alert in order to resolve complex mathematical relationships and there is no doubt that an active mind enjoys an exciting challenge in trying to make it intelligible. It likes complexity provided it can resolve it.

There is no doubt also that the reaction depends on a person's understanding of life and the world and that although repetitive monotony which deadens the activity of the brain may satisfy some, it will bore others.

The antiquity of music is not in question. Remains of men from thousands of years ago are sometimes accompanied by effective though primitive musical instruments like pipes or whistles. There is insufficient evidence to suppose they used more complex musical instruments but we are also unable to say for sure whether these primitive men could speak. It may be that music as a form of communication co-existed or even preceded the development of language itself.

Despite this, we do not know what makes a sound "musical". It was Pythagoras who pointed out that if two strings held at the same tension but of different lengths are plucked together they give a pleasant sound provided the length of the strings are in the ratio of two small integers. For instance if the lengths are in the ratio of 1:2 or of 2:3 they sound rather pleasant.

The sound made by the strings of ratio 1:2 is what we call an octave. We can say that a tenor and a soprano are singing the "same" note, even though they produce a very different frequency, provided they are in the same ratio. If the string is divided into three and the longer length, that is two-thirds, is plucked it gives us the "fifth". Division into four parts gives the "fourth".

Since the time of Pythagoras these intervals have been used formally and the basic scale of Western music is derived from the intervals of a tone and is therefore known as the *diatonic scale*. Pythagoras' discovery was one of the first examples of a numerical relationship in nature and was therefore of great significance to Pythagoras and his followers. They were so impressed with this idea that they gave these numerical relationships mystical meanings and believed that calculation of the sizes and orbits of the heavenly bodies would lead to similar discoveries. This was known as the "music of the spheres". The fact that music had often been associated with ritual and mysticism could only strengthen their beliefs, but the startling observation that Pythagoras had made was that a "pleasant" sound, one that gave rise to a good feeling, had a numerical basis.

Today we can both record and analyse sounds electronically and show the wave-form of the vibrations as a graph. We can demonstrate in that way the difference between a musical note and what we consider to be noise, a distinction we can make anyway just by listening.

A musical note could be very short like a piano note or it could be very long and sustained as when a wind instrument is blown. If we express it as a graph we will see that long or short, high or low, it has a periodicity and its shape will repeat itself again and again whereas the noise will be quite irregular and unrepeatable (Figure 21).

Things are, of course, never simple, and with experimental modern music attempting to use "non-musical" sounds as "music" our words

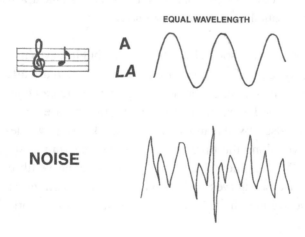

Figure 21. Sound of musical note compared to noise.

begin to lose their common meaning. Indeed John Cage, in his short piece *4'33"*, uses no sound at all. The pianist raises the piano lid and sits with his hands at the ready for four minutes and thirty three seconds. It is the pregnant silence in expectation, the tension in the audience waiting for a tone, the extraneous sounds of uneasy shifting and perhaps the odd suppressed cough that produces the emotion and is itself the performance. Calling this silence music, however, makes our use of words meaningfully difficult as they would require more elaborate definition.

For my purpose, the musical tone would have to be the one which provides the periodic repetition. Most musical instruments, however, vibrate in a manner more complex than simple repetition even though there is a repeat pattern.

There is always a fundamental frequency as in the pure tone, but there are also higher frequencies or overtones that we call "harmonics". These are integral multiples of the lowest or fundamental frequency and are in simple ratios such as 3:2 or 5:3 and so on. It is these higher harmonics that give a quality to a note which distinguishes one instrument from another.

When such musical intervals are produced in sequence they form a melody and in combination form harmony.

In his book *Theme and Variations* the violinist Yehudi Menuhin said:

> "Music creates order out of chaos; for rhythm imposes unanimity upon the divergent; melody imposes continuity upon the disjointed and harmony imposes compatibility upon the incongruous."[3]

It is in that way that sound becomes music, but it leaves us with two big questions: How do these combinations of sounds actually affect the brain itself? What is the nature of the messages that music can convey?

We have a good idea of how sound vibrations are transformed into electrical impulses by the inner ear and we know how these electrical impulses travel along the fibres of the nerve of hearing to special centres in the brain. We also know that at these centres the nerve fibres make connections with other nerves and so on. These connections are known as synapses and we now have quite a good idea how they work. It is by the

---

[3]Yehudi Menuhin, *Theme and Variations* (Stein and Day, New York: 1972).

release at the nerve ending of chemical substances that the receiving cell is stimulated into firing off new electrical impulses which travel on to the next one. Eventually they reach all sorts of different areas of the brain including part of the cerebral cortex and it is the activation of these cells which represents perception.

The mention of "chemical substances" today conjures up all sorts of thoughts and it is quite possible that when we say that a group of young people listening to extremely loud music and swaying with the beat appear to be "stoned" we are referring to the production of mood-changing chemicals in the brain as well as to the effect of substances which may have been ingested.

The description of the passage of impulses as being like the wiring of a house is too simplistic as nerve fibres in the brain are very numerous and travel to different centres at the same time. These centres or relay stations also receive many impulses from yet other areas of the brain so that in a way we can say that we may hear with the ear and appreciate what we hear with the whole brain.

There are differences, however. Dr Paul Broca had shown that speech was generally affected by lesions on the left side of the brain. Additionally there was the interesting case of a Soviet composer, Vissarion Shebalin, who had lost the use of language following a stroke affecting the left cerebral hemisphere. The Russian neuropsychologist Alexander Luria described how he was able to compose good music, despite the stroke. In his wonderful book, *The Man Who Mistook His Wife for a Hat*,[4] Oliver Sachs tells us about a musician who developed a rare neurological condition and, as a result, he could not even recognise simple objects. His understanding of music remained unimpaired however, and he used it to regain contact with the external world.

Studies of such patients have led to a general belief that the left hemisphere of the brain is analytical and logical, while the right is artistic. Even though this is an oversimplification, it does seem that the perception and processing of music as a received message is mainly located in the right hemisphere and language mainly in the left hemisphere.

---

[4] Oliver Sachs, *The Man Who Mistook His Wife for a Hat* (Gerald Duckworth & Co Ltd, London: 1985).

The second question is about the type of message that can be conveyed by music and the code by which the message is conveyed.

Whatever it is, the message must be more difficult to express in words, at least for some people, as otherwise that is how the message would have been presented. If music can communicate a feeling directly, what is it about a particular sound that will do this in a way that other sounds, such as those arranged as speech, or as noise, cannot?

Rhythm must have something to do with it. We are familiar with the effect of a marching drum-beat. For thousands of years men have advanced, shoulder to shoulder, to their deaths accompanied by the repetitive sound of the drums. At the other extreme, the pitch and its harmonics produced by the violin induce poignancy difficult to capture in words or even by other instruments although it can be achieved by the voice of good singers.

Creating order out of chaos induces serenity, and so sounds which are ordered and disciplined will give us a calming feeling. On the other hand we can also get bored and we require surprise, excitement and stimulus as well as serenity.

From time to time I hear broadcasts or recordings of music which had at one moment or another been disapproved of, scorned or even proscribed and I have always found it odd that authoritarians should care that much or should feel their power threatened by wordless music. The thought of Dmitri Shostakovich trembling with fear as Andrei Zhdanov attacked his music or when Joseph Stalin did not like his opera *Lady Macbeth of Mtebsk* left me puzzled. Why did they care so much as to consider killing a composer for music they did not like when they could simply not listen to it?

Clearly there must be something in common between the banned or censured pieces and we may well recognize it when we listen. Gypsy music can be delightful, sometimes sad, at times rousing and it is difficult to imagine why, like some of Shostakovich's music, it has ever been found threatening by authoritarian figures. It is likely that this fear is related to the lifestyle that it represents, which is communicated to us by sounds. The gypsy lifestyle may be dangerous, but there is something in it that we also crave; a certain lack of respect for constraint perhaps, a yearning to run away with the circus where no questions are asked as we move from place to place, away from parents, or indeed from children, as well as from authority. From time to time we may all want to dance with the wolves, but not all of the time, and perhaps we worry about our children doing so.

Many composers such as Johannes Brahms, Franz Liszt and Bedřich Smetana have included gypsy themes in their music, and by codifying them in a recognisable and repeatable form they have tamed them, so to speak, whilst still retaining much of their quality. It is curious that Klezmer music, which is related in some way to gypsy music, does not seem to have inspired the same type of threat.

In the same way, perhaps, jazz may have been tamed sufficiently by George Gershwin and Cole Porter to allow it to make the transition into our general culture of which it has become a part. Though now so familiar, it must have given a powerful message to cause it to be banned by the Nazis as well as by the Communists, and it is looked on with grave suspicion by Islamic regimes today.

The common denominator of those who banned jazz or gypsy music is control, authoritarianism and repression. The different types of disapproved music all show a certain loosening of rules, but it is not only in modern times that we have seen authority, religious or secular, feeling threatened by particular arrangements of musical tones. It may be that these authorities were right in their anxiety regarding the possible effects of music, although repression carries its own risk. In his play *The Bacchae* the ancient Greek playwright Euripides was very aware of the problem of excessive repression.

He has the well-meaning king, who sees it as his duty above all to keep the state safe and in good order for people to live without fear. However, he has to handle the arrival of a new cult. Belief in a new god, Bacchus, was spreading and he looked on the phenomenon as indeed we ourselves might — benignly if condescendingly. He himself cannot get involved but he does not see why it affects him or the state. Rumours that there is something improper about the cult soon begin to spread as it starts to get out of control and there are whispers of abandoned behaviour and even of sexual impropriety. Women appear to be the most affected, resulting, it is suggested, in the break up of families. Soon the rumours turn into formal complaints and the king is pushed into taking action to suppress the cult. In the process, the king is destroyed and Bacchus, or Dionysus as he was also known, takes his place among the established gods. The moral of the play is that there is a part of our nature that is wilder, looser and difficult to control, but it is there, and we cannot forcibly suppress it. If we do, we risk our own destruction. The only alternative, as Euripides saw it, is to accept the new god who also bears the name of "the loosener" and incorporate him into our culture. We should organise his rituals, sing his songs and pay homage to him during appropriately dedicated festivals. By recognising the uncontrollable we can contain it, bringing order out of chaos.

In a similar way, perhaps Gershwin sanitised jazz, leading it into our culture in an orderly manner, accepting that we need it. Perhaps Brahms and Liszt allowed us to enjoy gypsy music in a form which does not destroy our society and where we may not need to actually run away with the gypsies and dance with the wolves, but only to experience the feelings by listening to their music.

We are still left to wonder how exactly the message is transmitted from the feelings of the composer through the performer to his audience. Clues may perhaps emerge by looking back in history, but unfortunately we do not know what Greek music sounded like at the time of *The Bacchae*. Much less ancient Egyptian or Babylonian music, though Jewish psalms have probably contributed to the development of the music of our own time through early church hymns and plainchant.

We know that Pythagoras showed how intervals were used to produce musical sounds and that from these notes different modes were derived. They bore the names of the legendary Greek tribes: Dorian, Phrygian, Lydian, Aeolian and others and they seem to have been melodic formulae based on particular scales.

Aristotle tells us in his *Politics* that listening to the Mixo-Lydian mode made men mournful and solemn, whereas the Dorian strain relaxed them and made them good-tempered.[5] Indeed Plato, ever the authoritarian who favoured a strictly controlled society unacceptable to our Western liberal outlook, wanted to ban sad and plaintive music or music associated with drunkenness or laziness. The only two modes that he would allow in his

---

[5] Aristotle *Politics*: Book VIII, line 5–7.

Republic was the Phrygian and the Dorian, "the strain of courage and the strain of temperance" for war and peace.[6]

The Greek belief that music has an important effect on the soul and that it affects people's behaviour was reflected in their religion. There were two major cults, one centred on the god Apollo and the other following Dionysus, or Bacchus. They were not mutually exclusive and did not represent different religions. They are important to us because the different cultural strands that they highlighted have not ceased to exist through history and are certainly part of our lives today.

The Apollo cult expressed a classical approach to life. It was clear cut, objective and intellectual. It was associated with its own music and its principal instrument was the kithara, a form of lyre.

The romantics were devoted to Dionysus and favoured wind instruments. They approached life in a sensual and subjective way and their emotional abandonment both enriched Greek society and threatened to destabilise it and, indeed it still does, hence the "disapproved" music. It is interesting that it was most often associated with women; even now Orthodox Jewish synagogues shun women's voices in their choirs.

Deryck Cooke referred to "the language of music" suggesting that it must contain a message which can be followed from its conception by the composer to its effect on the listener. This way of looking at music is not universally accepted. Paul Hindemith, for instance, seems to have been irritated by the insistence that the composer has a message to convey. He says in his book *The Composer's World* that "music cannot express the composer's feelings...."[7] He gives the impression that he may just be composing in order to sell an interesting piece.

So much of what is written now is concerned with form, with intellectual analysis, with construction and is not intended to offer meaning. In many ways it resembles the visual culture of the 20th century, where message or even just content has been by-passed by interest in form as an abstract concept.

The question remains as to what it is in the actual sound that produces the different emotions. The major third can induce positive feelings like

---

[6]Plato *Republic*: Book III, line 398–403.
[7]Paul Hindemith, *The Composer's World* (Anchor Books, New York: 1961, p. 42)

joyful triumph, calm confidence, even love. It is present early in the harmonic series and may have been associated with the Ionian mode, where the major system was thought to be the basic harmony of nature.

We know this because that mode continued through the Graeco-Roman period and was widespread in medieval times in the songs of the troubadours. And yet, in 1322 Pope John XXII issued a decree (Papal Bull, *Docta Sanctorum*: 1323) banning the major third from church music as inappropriate except on special occasions stating that:

"… devotion, the true end of worship, is little thought of, and wantonness which ought to be eschewed increases … yet, for all this it is not our intention to forbid, occasionally and especially on Feast Days or in solemn celebration of the mass, the use of some consonances, for example the octave, fifth and fourth, which lighten the beauty of the melody…"

Rarely has there been such a precise indication of which sounds can have particular effects as this one, stated in the early years of the 14th century.

A one–two rhythm recalls the alternating steps of marching feet and it is not surprising that it is used in war to encourage the soldiers to march. Yet by the simple expedient of changing the rhythm to a one-two-three/one-two-three we can find ourselves dancing, whirling with abandon to the tempo of a waltz.

By going from the major to the minor key and by alternating the rhythm slightly the composer can play with our emotions even more than can be done with words.

The tritone interval, the sum of three whole tones which is also an augmented fourth, does not sound very pleasant and in the 13th century was referred to as *discordantia perfecta*. It was rejected as a consonance until the Renaissance and, as commonly happened, was even banned as *diabolus in musica*, because the devil was associated with chaos and discordance. It seems that as they understood that music creates order out of chaos and that the repetitions in tonal music give a sense of social order, they feared that dissonance might destroy the social order, leading to anarchy. This undermining of established concepts would be made worse as the absence of meaning in musical or literary form also frees the imagination which may in turn lead to another, very different, social order.

In time the tritone found a place as part of a progression and in 19th century romantic opera it often indicates evil, or at least the ominous; one example of this is in the dungeon scene of Act II in Beethoven's *Fidelio*. Dissonance has since been used extensively in film music where the ominous sound is not always perceived as demoniacal but instead carries a musical tension followed by release, put to good use by Igor Stravinsky in *The Rites of Spring*.

The essence of jazz is perhaps the despair and sadness which comes from slavery, but when intermixed with happiness and joy jazz becomes the blues. The result is a set of complex emotions, bitter-sweet and multi-faceted. My favourite is in West Side Story, when Leonard Bernstein introduces a dissonance interval in the most romantic and beautiful song, *Maria*.

6.3 Music and Deafness

I was once asked to give a talk at a music festival in Spoletto, Italy, as the organisers had decided to include a section on science and music. When I asked what they wanted of me they were vague: "You know, Beethoven's deafness. That sort of thing."

Every doctor with an interest in music and the history of medicine has speculated on Beethoven's illness. Every now and again there is a new book or article containing another suggestion or theory. In view of the prevalence of the condition at the time, syphilis is always blamed first but I feel, whether he had syphilis or not, that his many symptoms are not related to that disease. Otosclerosis has also been blamed with no good reason, as well as Pagct's disease, on the grounds that he had a rather large head in one of his portraits. There is really no way of knowing what the cause of his deafness was and I could not bear to waste everybody's time at the festival with yet another speculative list of differential diagnosis so I decided to talk about something quite different.

I put a lot of work into it and thought it had gone well. When the time for questions came a few hands went up. Every single one wanted my opinion on some aspect of Beethoven's illness though I had not even touched upon it.

It seems that there are really two questions which fascinate people. First, what was the cause of Beethovan's deafness? Second, how could he compose such extraordinary music when he could barely hear it or not at all?

He was not able to conduct adequately when he was very deaf and some of the saddest accounts are of his desperate attempts to conduct for as long as he could. He was unable to hear the tumultuous applause he received and he banged the piano oblivious to the discordant sounds he was producing.

As far as we are aware, there is no known family history of deafness. He came from a musical people as his father was a tenor in the Court choir and a singing teacher, while his grandfather had been the Kapellmeister or musical director at the Bonn Court of the Elector Maximilian Friedrich.

At the age of 26 he began to hear a buzzing tinnitus and to mishear words. After that the deafness got progressively worse, robbing him of much of the social and personal pleasures that his dominating position in music and ever-growing reputation should have afforded him.

In 1802, when he was only 32, he wrote to his brothers, Carl and Johann, a pathetically sad and frustrated letter: "You men who think or say I am hostile, peevish or misanthropic how greatly you wrong me." He went on to say that despite a temperament that enjoyed society, he had to withdraw himself and to spend his life alone. He told them how it was impossible for him to speak to people, always saying "Speak louder, shout, for I am deaf." He lamented:

> "How could I possibly admit weakness of the one sense which should be more perfect in me than in others, a sense which I once possessed in the greatest perfection, a perfection such as few in my profession have or ever have had?"

He was often near to suicide but he said it was impossible for him to leave this world "until I have produced all that I felt was within me…" He anticipated the need to understand his own illness as he added in his letter to his brothers the request that "as soon as I am dead, if Dr Schmidt is still alive, ask him in my name to describe my disease, and attach this written document to his account of my illness …"

Recently the writer Russell Martin told the story of how a lock of Beethoven's hair was acquired by two American admirers and subjected to DNA tests and other examination. The causes of his deafness still could not be decided but it was finally clear that it could not have been syphilis as no mercury was found in the hair. Mercury was the treatment for syphilis at the time, as well as for other infective diseases. They did, however, find an excessive amount of lead, enough to explain his various symptoms, though not his deafness. Lead poisoning was relatively common at the time as so many cooking utensils contained lead, and lead compounds were sometimes added to wine to sweeten it. Even then "plumbing" wine was known to cause colic.

Maybe one day, when new techniques are available, we will know the actual cause of Beethoven's deafness. More likely, however, we will be left to speculate on the more interesting and mysterious question of how a man so deaf for so long could compose music of such depth, each generation reviewing it in the light of its own experience and emotional needs.

It may be that, in the first place, the music is in the brain and the memory of the tones is enough to transpose and convert it into wonderful concepts and ideas. The rest depends on the strength and courage of Beethoven's own principles. His strong moral beliefs had led him to support Napoleon as the liberator of Europe and he composed his uplifting third symphony with the intention of calling it the *Bonaparte*. When his friend Ries told him in 1804 that his hero had proclaimed himself Emperor, he angrily tore up the title page of his manuscript crying,

"So he too is nothing more than an ordinary man. Now he will trample on all human rights and indulge only his own ambition. He will place himself above everyone else and become a tyrant."

Beethoven renamed his symphony the *Eroica*.

It may be that his misery, his courage and his capacity to overcome despair itself allowed him to convey his feelings to his fellow men in musical terms so powerful that what he produced has become one of the pillars of our culture. His is the finest example of a man successfully transmitting emotion in this way without the use of words.

The Czech composer Smetana also grew deaf, and during the final decade of his life he wrote a string quartet entitled *From My Life*, in which he very movingly portrays his growing deafness and the tinnitus that assailed him. He died in 1884 and it is know that syphilis was the cause.

I have from time to time listened to music on the radio or in the concert hall played by a soloist or a conductor, whose hearing I had tested and knew to be defective, and have been impressed by the beauty of the performance. I have records of the hearing levels of distinguished performers which show the inevitable changes of old age and yet I have felt that they had never played better. Anyone who has attended the 70th, 75th or 80th birthday performance of great musicians knows that the years have only added to the quality of their playing and yet there is no doubt that their hearing has deteriorated in the higher frequencies, just like that of everyone else. I once listened to one fine singer who had lost a great percentage of his hearing sing through a whole opera during which I am sure few had detected that he had a problem.

There are many elements involved in appreciating and performing music; deaf people, for example, can dance. Many dance very well as the rhythm of the music (which today is usually very loud anyway) can be felt in the vibrations of the floor, although some claim that they dance to an inner rhythm. In the early 1970s Cadillac Eddie and the Rabble Rousers, who were very deaf, were a perfectly reasonable rock band.

Deafness is not seen as a barrier to the enjoyment of music, so much so that the Mary Hare School, a residential school for deaf children in England, pioneered the teaching of music as part of its curriculum.

Many people who have a hearing loss worry about their future enjoyment of music. The majority will have mainly lost the higher frequencies, which seems not to impair the perception of music, although it can cause serious problems with the perception of speech.

Chapter 7

Poetry and the Sound of Words

Everyone knows what poetry is and yet it is difficult to define. Wordsworth said that it takes its origin from emotion recollected in tranquillity though some contemporary poets insist that they can only write in anger and in these cases the language is certainly intensified, as though highly charged. Much is made of its sensory, especially visual, images but the sound of the poem remains at its core.

> *Mais où sont les neiges d'antan*
> (But where are the snows of yesteryear)

The French poet François Villion was born in 1431, the year Joan of Arc was burnt at the stake. Inspired by the beauty of natural sights and sounds, the language he had to work with, the French of the time, was too poor to allow full scope to his feelings so he borrowed words from Latin and Greek as well as from old French. Most of all he looked for words which had a curious and interesting sound, taking them from slang, the jargon of the crafts, the jobs people did, from hunting and falconry. The sounds, their rhythms and cadences mattered very much, as most people were not able to read and could only listen to the poetry.

When I was 15 I left my home forever, though I did not know it at the time, and my mother gave me three tiny books of poems, one by François Villon, one by Pierre de Ronsard and the other by Joachim du Bellay.

I read them again and again even though I did not easily follow such old French. Yet the lines expressed sentiment just by their sound and brought back emotions that tied me to my family and my home. I recited the words of these men to myself seeking comfort mainly from the sound they made.

It was only much later that I learnt that both Ronsard and du Bellay had been deaf. Pierre de Ronsard had lost his hearing in his teens while Joachim du Bellay, his follower and admirer, became profoundly deaf through illness in his early 20s. Du Bellay wrote of Ronsard's deafness in one of his poems, reflecting that it may have protected him from irksome noises.

They were by no means the only profoundly deaf poets and clearly the memory of sound remains for them just as it did for Beethoven in his later compositions, and one wonders whether the silence can intensify the memory. Perhaps it allows the poet, like the musician, to explore it in ways that may have otherwise been overlooked.

Dorothy Miles, the poet who became deaf through meningitis, wrote of "the words and music that still sing in my mind." She tried also to blend words with sign language as closely as lyrics and tunes are blended in song so that it becomes reminiscent of mime.

There are also people who have never heard but have written wonderful poems, often with a searing visual imagery.

Often relegated to slim volumes in tiny corners of libraries the importance of poetry and poets continues to astound. These works have been preserved and treasured since antiquity and in our own time they are often the first to be banned by political oppressors. In some way the content, beliefs and hopes perhaps widely held and discussed, become more intense and urgent because of the language of poetry.

It has a special relationship with all the senses but most particularly vision and hearing, though now it is often the content that seems to be dominant. This may be because today we tend to read poetry silently rather than listen to it being declaimed out loud and the effect seems to be different. A friend who had never shown signs of being particularly poetic or spiritual confessed to the intensity of the feelings that had been generated towards his new love by reading poems to each other. He was so moved by the experience that he overcame his embarrassment in order to tell me that he had never known anything like it.

The French poet Arthur Rimbaud became so interested in the visual nature of poetry that he saw it as a form of synaesthesia. This is a curious effect, which some occasionally call a symptom when they find it disturbing, where one sensory stimulus produces a response in another sense. A sound, for instance, may induce a particular taste in the mouth or a smell.

Rimbaud tried to produce what he called "a systematic derangement of the senses" by finding colour in vowel sounds. "A" was black, for instance, "E" white, "I" red, "U" green and "O" blue. Not much came of this but it recalls the psychedelic experiments of the 1960s.

We cannot dismiss the visual experience — often by just looking at a sheet of writing without even reading it, in a foreign language perhaps, we are able to appreciate that the piece of writing is a poem.

The extent to which a poem depends on content remains uncertain. It may tell a story if it is in the narrative style or it could be purely descriptive. Very often it has a theme which may be an abstract way of representing a point of view or a philosophical approach but in the end poetry relies on the language and emotional implication of the words which the poet has chosen.

For example, the use of the word "slender" used in the context of a woman's "slender frame" is more emotionally charged in a love poem than describing her as having a "thin body". And yet in a doctor's case notes or in an article on starvation in a drought-ridden land a girl's "thin body" evokes the greater feeling. Here it is not so much the sound of the words which generates the emotion but some other quality, although the sounds of the words "slender" and "thin" may also have an effect.

The importance of the sound of language over content is expressed in Robert Frost's comment that "poetry is what gets lost in translation".[8] Yet most poetry is actually read in translation and enjoyed though the repeated attempts at new versions that each generation produces suggests that it is never entirely satisfactory.

Some say that poetry is simply another way of using language. Some even think it may have preceded prose and that it originates from the recitation of magical spells but there is no consensus. It may well be true, however, that the sound of the words directly affected the human spirit just

---

[8]Cleanth Brooks and Robert Penn Warren, *Conversations on the Craft of Poetry* (Holt, Rinehart and Winston: New York, 1959).

as the sound of music did before writing was invented, possibly even before spoken language as we know it evolved.

Poetry does not necessarily involve sound as a great deal of visual imagery emerges from similes, suitable epithets and especially metaphors.

7.1 Sound Patterns

Some of the earliest poems seem not to be concerned with sound at all, and biblical verses are said to be devoid of rhyme or metre and to rely on what has been called *semantic parallelism* where the lines of verse are parallel in meaning though not necessarily in sound. If the poet says "hearken" in the first verse he may say "listen" or "heed" in the second. One example of semantic parallelism is found in David's psalm (2 Samuel v22)

> For with you I charge a barrier
> With you I vault a wall.

I have never been convinced that this use of parallel meaning, which is complex and interesting, means that there was no use made of sound patterns as we cannot know what the phonetics of the period sounded like. The mere fact that lines of poetry are obviously recognisable even on the unread page suggests that its recitation involves stopping at intervals different from those of prose punctuation and that it could, if not should, be read differently.

When we look at the poem on the page it is usually divided into groups of lines rather than flowing continuously as in prose. These intervals provide a breathing space but it also groups together associated concepts and sounds. It is like a room or chamber and we can sit in it or walk about within its boundaries and then pass into another room in expectation and wonder, at least if the poem pleases or interests us. The word *stanza* to describe these groups of lines is from the Italian for room. At another level it stems from *stare* which means "to be located", and is related to *essere* which means just "to be", so that the implications get deeper and deeper.

The poet can decide how many lines he wants to put in his "room" or stanza as this has an effect both on the organisation of the images and on the sound and appears to inspire a particular feeling.

It is interesting that certain numbers have been especially popular. Four-line *stanzas* are called "quatrains" and are very common in English like Tennyson's *In Memoriam*:

> Calm and still light on yon great plain
> That sweeps with all its autumn bowers,
> And crowded farms and lessening towers,
> To mingle with the bounding main:

Groups of four or five can impose too much constraint on the poet for what he wants to say, imprisoning his mind. Shakespeare's sonnets are often 14 lines which has a totally different effect from that above.

Couplets, which are two-line *stanzas*, have a strangely liberating effect, with each *stanza* following its own idea. One fine example is the poem *Leisure* by W.H. Davies:

> What is this life if full of care,
> We have no time to stand and stare?
>
> No time to stand beneath the boughs
> And stare as long as sheep or cows.
>
> No time to see, when woods we pass,
> Where squirrels hide their nuts in grass.
>
> No time to see in broad daylight,
> Streams full of stars like skies at night.
>
> No time to turn at Beauty's glance,
> And watch her feet, how they can dance.
>
> No time to wait till her mouth can
> Enrich the smile her eyes began?
>
> A poor life this, if full of care,
> We have no time to stand and stare.

This was one of the first poems I learnt at school when recitation was rewarded. I had found the rhythm pleasing although the sentiments had little impact. After all, the metaphors and similes of nature and physical beauty did not impress a boy who was interested in tanks and guns, growing up as he was in the wartime.

When I recited the first line I had hooked on to a beat. There is, of course, a stress on the second syllable:

> What *is* / this *life* / if, *full*/ of *care*,
> We *have* / no *time* / to *stand* / and *stare*?

I recited the whole poem to the general hilarity of the class in this way:

> Ti-*Tum* / Ti-*Tum* / Ti-*Tum* / Ti-*Tum*

Though pleased with my showing off I realised it was not meant to be funny but fortunately we had a good teacher who entered the spirit of the thing by beating the rhythm with his ruler.

"Why don't you say 'What?' as though you are asking a question," he said. "And why not stop for a moment after the comma?"

> *What* is this *life*, … if *full* of *care*,

The beat, which gives rhythm to the verse, has to be subtle to be effective and not distort the language and make it sound ridiculous.

Many decades later I learnt that Mr Bullen, our teacher, had founded a literary and artistic magazine in Cairo during the Second World War and published Lawrence Durrell and many other writers as well as illustrators such as Edward Bawden.

In music we might say that there are four beats to each bar and therefore the "metre" is 4/4/. When this is the case we say that this poem is in "tetrameter" because it has four stresses per line.

Again, the poet does what he thinks will give the best results, and English poetry seems to be full of verses that are divided in fives which we call "pentameter", such as Oliver Goldsmiths' *The Village Preacher*:

> Near yonder copse where once the garden smiled
> And still where many a garden flower grows wild.

Hexameters, in sixes, were quite popular at one time and were called "alexandrines".

The stresses, although an integral part of the rhythm, can also be taken, in their own right, as part of the sound pattern.

Today, with attention being given mainly to content and to visual images, free verse has tended to degenerate into prose as concern with sound patterns have been pushed aside. Poetry has often become more prosaic, so to speak.

It is of course for the poet to offer what he can and for his public to like it or not. He may decide to insert monotonous prose into his poetry to achieve a particular effect or make a special point but, on the whole, most people respond to musicality in a poem and admire the poet's technique in orchestrating language as though it were a sort of verbal music. Jack Kerouac once noted in *Mexico City Blues* that he really wanted to write "like a jazzman blowing his horn and improvising."[9]

This musicality is acheived by using sound effects and it shares with music the rhythm and the beat that is built into it.

7.2 Rhythm, Beat and Metre

Ballads are actually songs that tell a story and that is where poems cross over into song and their sound can properly be called music. Traditionally a stanza is a quatrain with four beats in the first and third line and three in the second and fourth as in the traditional English ballad *Fair Margaret and Sweet William*

> There came a ghost to Margaret's door,
> With many a grievous groan;
> And aye he tirled at the pin,
> But answer made she none

On the other hand Keats achieves a very powerful effect in *La Belle Dame Sans Merci* by changing the stress in the last line of each stanza:

> O what can ail thee, knight-at-arms.
> Alone and palely loitering?

---

[9] Jack Kerouac, *Mexico City Blues*, note (Grove Press, New York: 1959).

> The sedge is wither'd from the lake,
> And no birds sing.
>
> O what can ail thee, knight-at-arms,
> So haggard and so woe-begone?
> The squirrel's granary is full,
> And the harvest's done.

In this poem the stress is placed on the second syllable and it is this that creates the metre or beat:

> O what can ail thee, knight-at-arms

This is very commonly used in English poetry and is called iambic metre. Indeed Shakespeare uses this beat so frequently that there is no better way to recognise it than to listen to his plays, for instance this passage from *The Merchant of Venice*:

> The quality of mercy is not strain'd
> It droppeth, as the gentle rain from heaven
> Upon the place beneath: it is twice blessed

There are five "iambs" to a line of verse and so it is called "iambic pentameter" and here it is not rhymed and therefore what we call "blank verse". By comparison, part of the effect in Keats' poem above is the variation in the beat in the last two syllables in the last line of each stanza, "… birds sing" and "… harvest's done" as they are equally stressed.

This equal stress is called a "spondee" as opposed to the iamb and the change in sound pattern has a marked effect on atmosphere.

Another way to change the sound pattern through a change in the stress is the "trochee" where the accent is on the first syllable and not on the second. Blake uses this in his poem *The Tiger*:

> Tiger! Tiger! Burning bright
> In the forests of the night,
> What immortal hand or eye
> Could frame thy fearful symmetry?

Here the trochee, with its repeated stress on the first syllable and the resulting pattern which the sound takes gives a sort of relentless feel to the poem which adds to its fearsomeness.

No one was more concerned with rhythm than Shakespeare. His words turn into music as his soft and hard consonants and the position of his vowel sounds form a melody and he uses the pauses that result from the rhythm to accentuate the thoughts and concepts he proposes. He discusses it amusingly but seriously in *A Midsummer Night's Dream*, when the country bumpkins decide to write a play and Bottom asks Quince to write a prologue. Quince says:

> "Well, we will have such a prologue;
> and it shall be written in eight and six".

But Bottom has other ideas:

> "No, make it two more; make it eight and eight."

However when Bottom is frightened as he finds things around him are magically changed — indeed his own head has been turned into that of an ass — he sings a pathetic little song about the familiar country things he knows.

> The ousel-cock so black of hue,
> With orange-tawny bill,
> The throstle with his note so true,
> The wren with little quill:

It has eight beats in the first and third line and three in the second and fourth just as Quince had said the prologue should be written.

This eight and six sound pattern may comfort him because it was the metre of so many country songs and ballads. He mentions also the plain-song sound of the hymns he sings in church.

> The finch, the sparrow, and the lark
> The plain-song cuckoo grey,
> Whose note full many a man doth mark,
> And dares not answer nay.

7.3 Rhyme

Nothing captures the essence of poetry like rhyme. Very small children are delighted by the repetition of the sound and this is why our favourite nursery songs are rhymed. This is the case in almost all languages as the children recognise the echo.

Twinkle, twinkle little star,	(a)
How I wonder what you are	(a)
Up above the world so high	(b)
Like a diamond in the sky.	(b)

Here the end of each line rhymes with the next as in the sequence *aabb*.

In the French rhyme *Le Corbeau et le Renard* by Jean de la Fontaine the rhyme follows an *abab* pattern:

> *Maitre Corbeau, sur un arbre perché,*
> *Tenait en son bec un fromage.*
> *Maitre Renard, par l'odeur alléché*
> *Lui tint a peu près ce langage.*

However, rhyme has not always been in fashion. Ancient Greek and Latin poets do not appear to have relied on rhyme as they used metre to create their sound patterns. Ancient Chinese poetry used rhyme according to the tone patterns.

In time, some of the late Latin hymns began to rhyme, but it was the troubadours of the Middle Ages who really made a great deal of it in their poems of courtly love.

Since then it would be difficult to exaggerate the importance of rhyme in poetry and for many they have been synonymous. The echoes present in rhymes give a resonance to the sound when we read a poem aloud, and it introduces a sense of order. In looking for sounds which rhyme the poet is required to search for interesting and lesser known words in the language and as a result obscure words are brought to the fore. Rhyme also has a mnemonic quality which drives the poem deep into our minds.

In our early days as medical students we used such devices to remember our anatomy:

> The lingual nerve, it took a turn
> Around the hyoglossus
>
> After that it twists round Wharton's Duct, through which
> the saliva flows which said:
>
> The bugger's double crossed us!

It was not a very good poem and obviously after years of familiarity with the operative anatomy I do not need to use such tools for memory, but still the poem remains with me! There were many such rhymes that helped force anatomy into our memory, most of them, in the medical student style, too rude to repeat.

On the other hand, rhyme can be trite and sound funny in the wrong context. Isak Dinesen in *Out of Africa* said that her African workers called rhyming "speaking like rain" and that it made them laugh.

Certain rhymes can be funnier than others, for instance many feel that three syllable rhymes are funny. Byron uses these in his long and mocking poem *Don Juan*:

> And rash enthusiasm in good so/ci-e-ty
> Were nothing but a moral ine/bri-e-ty

and

> Without our knowledge or our *approba-ti-on*
> Although they could not see through his disguise,
> All felt a soft kind of *concatena-ti-on*.

Another appropriate and quite unexpected example of the comic quality of rhyme came with the arrival in the post of the *GKT Gazette*. *GKT* stands for Guy's, King's and St Thomas' as the three medical and dental schools have now amalgamated and are attempting to marry their considerable apocryphal traditions without losing them in the process. Among these are the numerous stories relating to John Keats, as he had studied medicine at Guy's and is commemorated by a wing which has been named Keats' House (though not everyone there realises that it refers to the poet). He was a very able and successful student and was offered a career as surgeon which he turned down as he wished to devote himself entirely to poetry. The June 2004 issue of the *Gazette* carried an interesting feature which told of Keats' classmate, Henry Stephens who was himself soon to invent the famous blue–black ink, and who had kept some lines which Keats had scribbled on the cover of his friend's chemistry notes:

> Give me women, wine and snuff
> Until I cry out "hold, enough!"
> You may do so sans *objection*
> Till the day of *resurrection*;
> For, bless my beard, they aye shall be
> My beloved Trinity.

In order not to be trite, of course, rhyme has to be interesting and new, otherwise it is better to do without. Most of the lines in Shakespeare's plays were written in blank verse; in this way the words did not constrain the flow of his imagination. On the other hand his sonnets would not be sonnets without rhyme;

> Love's not Time's fool, though rosy lips and cheeks
> Within his bending sickle's compass come;
> Love alters not with his brief hours and weeks,
> But bears it out even to the edge of doom.

Alexander Pope used a rhyming ten-and-ten to describe the deeds of heroes, *aabbcc* and so on and as a result this sound is known as the "heroic couplet". He shows this best in the combat between Hector and Ajax in his rendering of the *Iliad*.

> Now Ajax braced his dazzling armour on,
> Sheathed in bright steel the giant warrior shone;
> He moves to combat with majestic pace:
> So stalks in arms the grisly god of Thrace.

On the other hand Pope was well aware of how ridiculous this "heroic" couplet of rhymed iambic pentameter can be in the wrong context or if it is exaggerated.

In *The Rape of the Lock* Pope makes direct use of the same rhymed iambic pentameter to convey sarcasm in the narrative regarding the rather silly efforts of the hero to steal a lock of hair from his sleeping girlfriend:

> So ladies in romance assist their knight,
> Present the spear, and arm him for the fight.
> He takes the gift with reverence, and extends
> The little engine on his fingers' ends.

7.4 Onomatopoeia

Here words actually sound like the action they represent. For instance the word "splash".

I tried, as a test though admittedly using gestures as well, to indicate "splashing" to a non-English speaker who understood at once.

It is not surprising that such sounds have found their place in poetry as in Ted Hughes *The Wild Duck*:

> Through the precarious crack of light
> Quacking Wake Wake

7.5 Alliteration

Repetition of the initial consonant requires a nimbleness of tongue which generates interest as well as a suggestion of cleverness in its construction. Here is Gerald Manley Hopkins in *The Windhover*:

> I caught this morning morning's minion, kingdom
> of daylight's dauphin, dapple-dawn-drawn Falcon,
> in his riding.

This tongue-twister quality can also be used to create the absurd as in the French poem by Jacques Prevert:

La pipe au pape Pie pue

Tennyson found that he had to control himself as he had a natural tendency to alliterate his lines excessively and unwittingly.

Ancient English and Anglo-Saxon poetry relied almost entirely on alliteration as in Beowulf or in William Langland's *Piers Ploughman* which starts:

In a summer season when soft was the sun.

Contemporary poets seem to feel that they have to be careful with this sound pattern and there are also other considerations such as the time between each repeated consonant as the mind forgets the first if it is too far ahead.

The effect is more noticeable if repeated three times rather than only two, appearing more intentional, as though making a point. When I called my wife on her mobile telephone and she said she was in a queue "buying bagels", it was heard as a statement of fact and meant nothing more. However, if she were to add an alliterative adjective: "buying bloody bagels", her irritation shows not only by the irreverent adjective but also because of the relentless repetition of the initial consonant. It was an irritated *sound* that I heard. It was not meant to be a poem, of course, but she was showing her feelings and emotions.

While poets now tend to beware of too much alliteration, it is very popular with the advertising industry, as it shares with rhyme the capacity to insert itself into the memory.

7.6 Assonance

Assonance is related to alliteration but is the repetition of vowel sounds rather than consonants.

As vowel sounds are formed by the same range of frequencies that we find in music, the musicality of a poem is strongly affected by the way

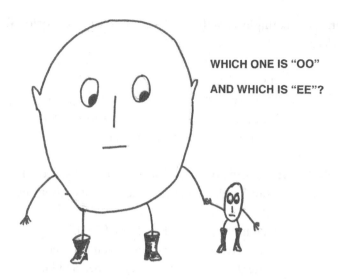

Figure 22. Oo-oo and Ee-ee.

these are arranged and they can provide a melody. Vowel sounds range from the low-pitched "oo" to the middle range "ah" and to the high-pitched "ee". These pitches indicate other qualities as well as introducing music.

One experiment that I carried out with small children when I held a hearing and language clinic at Guy's Hospital, was to show them cards with the two figures I had drawn (Figure 21). I told them that one was called "ee-ee" and the other "oo-oo" and asked them which they thought was which. All said that the big one was "oo-oo" and they were convinced that the little one was "ee-ee".

If we associate low pitches with bigness and high pitches with smallness we can introduce yet another subtle qualitative symbol into a poem simply by the use and arrangement of particular vowels.

The English language contains plenty of vowel sounds giving us many possibilities, though most of them are *diphthongs*. This is different from French and Italian, where the long and short pure vowels predominate. Diphthongs are complex vocalised sounds like "ai", "oi", "ia" or "ow".

Modern poets have found a way of avoiding what they feel to be the worst excesses of rhyme by changing the vowel in the rhyming syllable while maintaining the consonants and thus not losing the rhyme altogether. One example is Wilfred Owen in his First World War poem *Strange Meeting*:

> It seemed that out of battle I *escaped*
> Down some profound dull tunnel, long since *scooped*
> Through granites which titanic wars had *groined*.
> Yet also there encumbered sleepers *groaned*.

And so this moving poem goes on, with "bestirred" rhymed with "stared", "hall" with "Hell", "hair" with "hour" right down to its unsettling end:

> I am the enemy you killed, my friend.
> I knew you in the dark; for so you frowned
> Yesterday through me as you jabbed and killed.
> I parried; but my hands were loath and cold.
> Let us sleep now …

These imperfect or approximate rhymes are useful because English lacks rhyming words compared with many languages such as Italian or French, so this sort of rhyming offers us a "better than nothing" factor. Nevertheless, the rhymes are also pleasing, because the slight distortion of the sound pattern creates an element of surprise. The vowel is needed as the musical aspect of the verse but the poet or song writer can afford to change the consonant without affecting the music.

7.7 The Sound of Poetry

Sound plays an enormous part in poetry and when we look back at poetry through time and the role that metre, rhyme and the patterns of onomatopoeia, alliteration, the assonance and the music of the vowels plays, we see that their importance has varied with the generations. The reasons for this are complex, and may result from the continuous changes in our own language which bring in new words and unfamiliar sounds, the simple excitement of fashion and even new technological discoveries, such as the electronic technologies that have influenced music and which can be extended to poetry.

To be fashionable appears to be such a basic human need in every sphere from clothing, handbags and shoes to art, medicine, music; we can only be expected to welcome fashion in poetry too. The fact that changing fashions often generates such fury in those who feel threatened by change, no matter how temporary or trivial it is — even the shaving of beards or the playing of music can be repressed by massacres — testifies to fashion's extraordinary symbolic value.

I do not think there is a better explanation of intention than that in Vladimir Mayakovsky's poem *The 150,000,000,* published in 1921. Lenin thought it was stupid and pretentious and even Boris Pasternak did not think much of it. Here is the first stanza of the poem:

> We will smash the old order
> wildly
> we will thunder
> a new myth over the world.
> We will trample the fence
> of time beneath our feet.
> We will make a musical scale
> of the rainbow.

I am not sure what to make of this now but it is the translation by Anna Bostock and it brings back memories of visiting her at her house in Hampstead when I was a very young man. I remember little other than the fact that all the people there, artists and writers for the most part, called her "Anya", in the Russian manner, and that the conversation was of ideas and concepts. I do recall the feeling though, my breast beating with the excitement of changing the world with words and thoughts.

Today, the role of content, which is often political or some sort of social critique, seems to predominate in favoured poems and is enhanced by the powerful presence of visual images while intellectual exercise is demanded by the meditative poems brought about by the popularity of Zen *koans* which are supposed to set the mind free, such as the often quoted:

> "What is the sound of one hand clapping?"

We can invent many answers to that if we wish to play at philosophy, and one of these could be simply "nothing!" On the other hand I wonder what those who like mental puzzles would make of the sound pattern of a similar idea:

"The soulful song of the single silent slap".

Those who meditate sometimes use the resonating voiced "Om" together with contemplation and it seems that the vibration which spreads from the chest to the rest of the body helps to create a particular state of mind. Similarly, the combination of a sound which tends to make us feel sad with a sad thought has been common in songs and more recently in the music of films. In films, frightening music can enhance fearsome visual images. On the other hand, paradox (where the music does not match the emotion of the words or vice versa) can also have a special impact. Indeed, it is a peculiar aspect of Latin American music that very sad lyrics may be set to bright and happy sounding tune and the reverse.

Alexander Pope showed that the same can be done in poetry, as evident when he put the words of *The Rape of the Lock* into the heroic-sounding couplets he had used in his poetic translation of the tragic and grand battle between Hector and Ajax, taken from the *Iliad*.

It would be a pity if, as a result of being overwhelmed by content and visual image and shamed by the unfashionable position of metre, rhyme and sound effects such as alliteration, our children lost the pleasures of reciting poetry.

Part IV
Impaired Communication

To communicate using speech we need not only to be able to hear but also to have heard speech during the early, formative period of our childhood. Our brains need to be able to process what we hear and we also need to be able to pronounce the words we wish to express.

To hold a successful conversation using speech we have to be able to hear the sounds and differentiate between them in order to understand what they mean. We also have to have the ability to remember what has already been said.

When we speak we have to use proper words and to put them in a proper order. This process, which seems simple enough, is actually very complex and requires what are known as semantic and syntactic skills. Additionally, our motor system has to be functioning well enough for us to articulate our speech. Furthermore, some social skills are also needed as what we say has to be relevant and acceptable to our listener. To communicate using speech we need not only to be able to hear but to have heard speech during the early, formative period of our childhood. Our brains need to be able to process what we do hear and we also need to be able to pronounce intelligibly the words we wish to express. If we are not able to do this our capacity to communicate is impaired even though we can hear.

Despite this, language as a means of communication need not be expressed only by speech, as we also use gesture, touch, facial expression, eye contact and direction of gaze.

Communication is of course difficult when we are not able to hear as our society generally depends on sound. The problem has been overcome, first by using sign language and later with devices that amplify sound and procedures such as direct electrical stimulation of the cochlea.

Chapter 8

When Hearing is Impaired

There is a major difference between those who are deaf from birth or a very young age and those who became deaf after speech has been acquired.

An adult who has become deaf finds communication by speech difficult only because he cannot hear what is being said to him. He may acquire hearing aids, lip-read, and write notes, but his own capacity to communicate is unimpaired as he can speak when he wishes to express himself. If he is profoundly deaf, the quality of his own speech may alter, but not enough to be incomprehensible.

It is quite different when a person is deaf from birth as, if he has never heard the sounds of speech, he cannot reproduce them, so that speaking may be very difficult or impossible. This is why we are so concerned with the education of the deaf child, as, unless it is undertaken at an early age, failure to educate them correctly may mean failure to give the child a chance to speak.

This chance is provided by the early use of hearing aids and, more recently, the introduction of cochlear implants, but mainly by special education, an arduous enterprise for everyone concerned, child, parents and teacher.

8.1 Two Approaches

There have been opposing attitudes towards profoundly deaf children. Should they be left to communicate among themselves with their hands? Should parents of deaf children accept that they belong to another perfectly respectable but separate community? Or should we see our deaf children as suffering from a disability that we should mitigate as much as possible, tethering them to ourselves as tightly as we can?

A third, fuzzier way relies on doing the best we can in each case which, although it seems the most reasonable, leaves a lot to be desired as our best is not always good enough.

In 1976 I presented my work on the cochlear implant to the Royal Society of Medicine in London, receiving a standing ovation from my fellow surgeons and what I had to say was reported in the press as a "bionic ear" for the first time. Progress, however, turned out to be slow and not always backed by the encouragement which that reception had led me to expect.

The criticism was because we could still not restore normal hearing and some believed that if it did not cure deafness completely our work had no place at all.

Parents of deaf children often found it difficult to come to terms with their plight despite great efforts by deaf support groups to help them accept signing. Many feared that the allure, distant or not, of a bionic ear would prevent acceptance and it was better for us not to upset people with dreams of a future that was not for them.

Walking to a conference in Manchester I saw a demonstration and there were people holding placards that said:

"LEAVE THE DEAF ALONE"

Some carried my name but inside the hall there was great interest in our work and it was only when questions were invited that I sensed any hostility. A deaf man who had no speech, sent up a note which was read out by the chair, herself the mother of two deaf girls. Its words still affect me:

"Tell him to leave the deaf alone. They have their own language and their own culture. To try and put an end to it is a form of cultural genocide."

Research is difficult and dogged with failure, while any returns are slow to come by, and ours was only an episode in an enterprise over many years. Another event also took place at a meeting of experts from all over the world, in Paris this time, when we sat in the ancient Cathedral of Notre Dame waiting for a concert to begin. Around me were many who had given most of their lives to help the deaf in one way or another, collected in the great nave, when the musicians began to play.

Suddenly they were interrupted by piercing whistles as people held up the placards which by now had become familiar to all of us from America to Australia, from France to Japan:

"LEAVE THE DEAF ALONE"

There was not much we could do and there was no one prepared to discuss it with us so we filed out quietly and went on our way.

8.1.1 *Sign Language*

In Paris there is an ancient street called Rue de l'Abbé de l'Épée. This strange name, translated as "The Street of the Priest of the Sword", suggests a crusader knight but it was in fact the name of a teacher of the deaf who had lived in the 18th century.

The Abbé de l'Épée, the son of a well-to-do architect, was a humble man who had decided at 17 to become a priest. "God has done everything for my welfare and I have done nothing in return for the excellence of his grace," he is often quoted as saying, but he also had an independence of spirit and a wish to help the underdog which would cause trouble with the Church establishment.

An obscure sect in the French Catholic church created a significant and dangerous controversy at the time. They were called Jansenists, after their founder Cornelius Jansen, and their beliefs involved predestination and denial of free will as well as hostility to the Jesuits. The young Abbé refused on principle to take an oath rejecting their teachings when he took holy orders.

The bishop of Troyes ordained him anyway, though he was not allowed to administer the sacraments and, considered too unsound for pastoral work, he remained an outsider in the eyes of both the Church and the State as Jansenism eventually became illegal.

Living in Paris on a family allowance, he wore clerical dress though he had no formal church position and spent his time helping the poor. Perhaps he saw the deaf as fellow outcasts, excluded as he was, from the usual activities of the church.

Among those he visited in the poor district of the Fosses-Saint Victor were a widow and her deaf twin daughters who made a living from sewing. The girls could not speak, read or write as deaf children did not go to school, though what really worried the Abbé was that, with no knowledge of Christianity and unable to take communion, the next world might be closed to them.

The Church followed St Paul's belief of *ex auditum fidem* or "faith comes through hearing": that it was only through the words of a preacher who taught the beliefs of the Church as established by the King could God be contacted.

Science hardly offered an alternative view as the philosopher Étienne de Condillac himself, whose influence was considerable, believed that abstract thought as well as memory required the symbols of language which were unavailable to the deaf. He eventually changed his mind, however, when he finally saw what the Abbé de l'Épée's deaf pupils were capable of.

When he began teaching the girls, the Abbé, too, believed that they had no language because they had no speech and as yet no one had made the distinction between the two. He thought that he would teach them writing first as he could show them an object and then write its name, though God, his real interest, was an abstract idea.

He soon realised that the girls had a language of their own, communicating feelings such as sadness and happiness between themselves by using hand signals as well as facial expressions and body movements. He thought that if he learned their language he could teach them to read and write French by signing and in that way give them religion.

The Abbé de l'Épée's wish to help those he felt were outsiders like himself, and his willingness to accept that it was he who had to do the learning, is what started the education of the deaf and his success caused great excitement throughout the world. The number of pupils grew, and his school in the Rue des Moulins held open sessions inviting visitors in order to gain support. The Abbé also held a mass in sign language at the church of Saint-Roche which the authorities did not prevent.

Queen Marie-Antoinette took her brother Joseph II, the Emperor of Austria, to observe the teaching. He was so impressed that he sent the Abbé Storck to learn the method and open a school in Vienna, while the Empress Catherine of Russia sent her ambassador. Scientists and philosophers came including Lord Monboddo who had interviewed the wild boy, Peter, and Memmie Le Blanc. De Condillac, who had previously stated that those devoid of speech could not have ideas, was so impressed that he not only changed his views, but now felt that sign language was less ambiguous than speech.

On his deathbed the Abbé de l'Épée received a delegation from the National Assembly of the new republic who had come to let him know that his school would continue under its auspices. The Abbé Sicard took over and the school moved to the Rue Saint Jacques (which is incidentally where Itard was to find the wild boy of Aveyron).

The Abbé de l'Épée was buried in the crypt of the church of St Roche, taking his place among the remains of other great men such as Denis Diderot, Pierre Corneille and Andrè le Nôtre.

The Convention, which had taken over from the Assembly, held hearings on the education of the deaf, though one representative claimed it was a waste of money to support the school as signing was widely used among deaf people without expensive training. Mistaken as this is, it shows how far the world had come in accepting that sign language had all the attributes of other languages as well as the parsimonious nature of parliamentary government.

The method of signing as a means for education deaf people reached the United States (in the early 19th century) before it came to Britain. It began with the education of a deaf girl, Alice Cogswell, who was born to a respected patrician family in Hartford, Connecticut. It was their neighbour, Thomas Gallaudet, who took on Alice's education and would eventually become responsible for the schools for the deaf in the United States.

Gallaudet was descended from the Huguenots, who wcre Protestants and had the same desire to do good as the Catholic Abbé de l'Épée. Gallaudet received financial support from both the Cogswells and his own family to go to Paris to learn the Abbé's method of teaching the deaf.

Gallaudet brought a deaf teacher, Laurent Clerc, from Sicard's school in Paris, thus initiating the teaching of the deaf by the deaf themselves using signing only. Since the signs had little to do with a particular language there were no problems with learning from a French teacher. Together Clerc and Gallaudet co-founded the first school for the deaf, with Gallaudet as the first principal.

Half a century after Gallaudet's school was opened in Hartford, Connecticut, Amos Kendall, a philanthropic businessman, gave some land for a school for the deaf and blind in Washington, D.C. He appointed Thomas Gallaudet's son Edward as headmaster with Sophia Fowler, Edward's mother, as matron.

The school thrived under Edward Gallaudet, who, like his father, appointed deaf teachers trained in sign language. The school was aimed at higher education and, in 1864, Congress authorised the institute as a national college. In time, a teacher training department was also set up at Gallaudet College and distinguished teachers have continued to graduate ever since.

The College eventually became a university, and still operates as such, with programmes in both arts and sciences. The university claims that 96% of its graduates enter full time employment or enrol for advanced studies and most of its students receive financial aid. The university remains committed to sign language, providing a unique community where the deaf and the hard of hearing as well as those who can hear, work together and enjoy a social life in an environment where communication is conducted entirely by signing.

8.1.1.1 *Sign languages around the world*

Signing depends on identifying visual rather than acoustic patterns and sign language uses body movements and position as well as facial expression although meaning is chiefly conveyed with the hands.

There are many sign languages and most countries have their own although these need not be related to the spoken language. There are some unexpected results: Britain and America, for instance, share the spoken English language, but they have distinct sign languages. American Sign Language (ASL) is derived from the old French Sign Language developed by the Abbé de L'Épée and is therefore distinct from British Sign Language (BSL) which was developed completely separately.

There is evidence of British signing since at least 1570 but it was first codified at Braidwood's Academy for the Deaf and Dumb in 1760 to become the "combined system" from which BSL is derived. The London Asylum for the Deaf and Dumb in Grange Road, Bermondsey, the first public educational institution for deaf children in England, was founded in 1792 and its first headmaster had been trained at Braidwood's.

Thomas Gallaudet had come to Britain on his trip to learn how to teach the deaf but he was badly received by the Braidwood schools. He went on to Paris where he was welcomed at the school in the Rue St Jacques. As a result, deaf Americans are more likely to be able to have a more intelligible conversation in sign language with a deaf French person than an Englishman using BSL. Similarly, a deaf American can converse better with a deaf person from Timbuktu because of its French connection.

Sign languages descended from BSL include those used in Australia, India and New Zealand. Indeed, I still find it strange that South Africa has 22 languages of which 11 are official, but all sign in BSL.

Other oddities illustrate how sign language has evolved. Chinese Sign Language (CSL) was invented by an American woman called Nellie Thompson Mills, the wife of a missionary. It is split into two dialects, a southern one centred on Shanghai which subsequently spread to Hong Kong and Singapore, and a northern one centred on Beijing. They are quite unrelated to Taiwanese sign language which is part of the Japanese family as it began to spread under Japanese rule.

A school using German Sign Language was established in Jerusalem by German immigrants in the 19th century, but after the Second World War the large number of immigrants who brought their own sign languages had to converse in a pidgin which evolved into a creole and has now become Israeli Sign Language, a language used by Muslims, Christians, Druze and Bedouin alike.

Attempts to have a unified Arabic Sign Language have failed as yet and the usual oddities exist as Moroccan Sign Language is related to ASL while Tunisian Sign Language is closer to Italian Sign Language. Egyptian Sign Language is on its own.

8.1.1.2 *How sign language works*

Although deaf people have always communicated by signs, it was in 1620 that a manual was published by Juan Pablo Bonet in Madrid, a book that had considerable influence in Europe and which used gestures as phonemes and contained a manual alphabet.

Sign language is not mime and linguistically it is as rich and complex as any spoken language leading to an even greater connection between form and meaning. Its grammar allows both concrete and abstract expression.

Where speech organises meaningless sound units or *phonemes* into meaningful semantic units the gestural equivalents act similarly and, although for a while known as *cheremes*, are now also called phonemes.

Sign language involves a number of elements called *tab*, *dez* and *sig*.

Tab: location of the hand (for instance, in ASL there are 12 hand locations).
Dez: the shape made by the hand.
Sig: is the motion carried out.

In addition to hand movements, facial expression is also used as well as mouthing and body posture such as raising the eyebrows to indicate a question.

ASL grammar has been the one most studied and has shown how *compounding*, that is combing the sign for *face* with that for *strong* becomes *resemble* whereas mouthing modifies words and adjectives. Repetition is also meaningful as repeating the sign for *chair* to indicate *sit*.

Generally, all sign language is constructed as *subject/verb/object* and relative clauses are indicated by tilting the head, raising eyebrows and the upper lip.

In these global times there is now an International Sign Language (IS) sometimes known as *Gestuno*. It is a sort of pidgin with a limited vocabulary; role playing seems to be quite important.

8.1.2 *Finger spelling*

Finger spelling is not a sign language nor, indeed, a language at all. It seems to have always been around and may have been used for calculation in the ancient Middle East where letters were often substitutes for numerals. The monks who had taken vows of silence are thought to have communicated in that way but today it is widely used by the deaf where there is no sign for a word, for instance in names of people or of products. Some people are very quick and are said to express the whole alphabet in less than 6 seconds. At a Hot Fingers competition held in England the speed was so great that the judges had to rely on slow motion film.

BSL uses two hands for the alphabet whereas most others, including ASL, use one.

8.1.3 *Hoping to speak*

The old city of Paris and its crowded, narrow streets was, in the 19th century, to be criss-crossed by wide Boulevards, busy with traffic and commercial activity. The French have no inhibitions about honouring their great men and recall their contributions by naming streets and thoroughfares after them. Like Rue de l'Abbé de l'Épée, Boulevard Péreire has an interesting place in our story.

The Péreire family have contributed so much to their country that the honour could apply to any one of them and for many deeds. Jacob-Emile and Isaac Péreire were among the first to establish the railway system in France and were also followers of the philosopher Saint-Simon in his support of social regeneration. Born during the Napoleonic Wars and growing up with great concern for the plight of the deprived, they had both been elected deputies to the National Assembly. Isaac's son Eugene was also elected to the National Assembly in 1863, around the time Gallaudet's college received the blessing of the Congress of the United States.

Part of Eugene Péreire's philanthropic project was to set up a whole system of schools for the deaf. However, unlike that of the Abbé de l'Épée and Thomas Gallaudet, he was committed to teaching the deaf to speak rather than to communicate only by signing. He believed the deaf to be among the most deprived, but he set up the schools in honour of his own grandfather Jacob Rodrigues Péreire.

Like the Abbé de l'Épée, Jacob Péreire was an outsider, but of a different kind. His family were Spanish Jews at a time when, under the rule of Ferdinand and Isabella, they were expelled from their homes and their country. The Pereira family fled to Portugal but to no avail as persecution followed them and, unable to flee yet again as conversion to Christianity in Portugal was enforced on the penalty of death, they returned to Spain.

Abraham Rodrigues and Abigail Rebecca Pereira were forced to convert publicly, to change their names to Juan and Leonora and their son, Jacob Rodrigues, was baptised Francisco-Antonio in 1715, the year Louis XV came to the throne of France.

Persecution continued anyway as the Inquisition was set up to root out any recidivists among the New Christians and almost 2,000 desperate converts were burned alive, accused of being secretly Jewish.

There was no respite for the Pereira family as Abigail, now widowed with several children, was accused of heresy. They managed to flee to France where Jewish refugees were tolerated in Bordeaux provided they paid 110,000 *livres* to the crown each time a new king succeeded.

The young Jacob Rodrigues Pereira reverted to his true name, though Pereira changed to Jacob Rodrigue Péreire as it was more easily pronounced by the French. But the survivors of the family faced another problem because Jacob's beloved sister was profoundly deaf.

Not yet 19, Jacob wrote to the president of the *Academie des Lettres* of Bordeaux to ask for a list of books on educating the deaf. His first pupil was his sister.

His success in getting her to speak led to an apprentice tailor aged 13 who had very little hearing and no speech, being brought to him and soon the boy was able to say a number of words. A nobleman, Monsieur d'Etavigny, who had a deaf son called Azy, heard about it and although this boy was now 18 and could read and write, he could not speak a word. Monsieur d'Etavigny, however, was not happy at the thought of entrusting the education of his son to a Jew, so he asked Péreire to write to the prior of the Abbey where Azy was a pupil, with details as to how he should be taught. The prior did not think he could handle the method and Jacob entered into a strange contract as he was to go to the Abbey where, in the presence of the priest, he was to teach the boy and be paid according to the number of words he learnt.

The results were so dramatic that the prior, a man of science, called together the *Academie Royale des Lettres* of Caen to observe what had happened and Azy addressed the bishop, to everyone's amazement, saying quite clearly: *"Monseigneur, je vous souhaite le bonjour!"*, which means "My lord, I bid you good day!"

Jacob Péreire moved to Paris, where he was already well known as the newspapers had picked up the story. The *Académie des Sciences* had publicly interviewed Azy and it is recorded that he spoke slowly but clearly and was able to answer questions. They were so impressed that a commission was set up to study Péreire's work and Comte de Buffon, the chairman, who was then writing his *Natural History of Man*, included Péreire's attainment in his famous book.

Péreire, together with Azy, were eventually presented to the King. The two outsiders stood in front of Louis XV, the most powerful man in Europe: Jacob Rodrigue Péreire, the Jew who had fled from country to country, and Azy d'Etavigny the boy excluded by his peers because he could not speak their language.

"Sire," Azy said. "I deeply appreciate the honour of appearing before Your Majesty."

Jacob Péreire was given an income by the King and taught many pupils. He became a friend of Denis Diderot and other intellectuals of the Enlightenment and, a true man of his time, he studied every aspect of science, making a calculating machine and writing a useful book about sail power.

He used any method he could, including hand signals, as his successful pupils probably had some residual hearing and some may well have been deafened after they had been exposed to speech. He encouraged sign language for the very profoundly deaf though many of his pupils were able to communicate by speech and lip-reading.

Despite it all, he was not allowed to open a school as the church would not let education of any sort be taught by a Jew, so the only public education provided for deaf children was that taught by the priests who never offered the possibility of speech, even to those who might perhaps have benefited.

When conditions changed and he could at last openly call himself a Jew, the first record of an application for permission for a Jewish cemetery in France is from Jacob Rodrigues Péreire.

When I started my clinic for children with hearing and language problems at Guy's Hospital I did not know who Péreire was although I had roamed along Boulevard Péreire in Paris in my teens. I was also unfamilier with the Braidwood School, which I was once asked to attend. Set up by the Inner London Education Authority, the school was responsible for deaf children below school age. Its work was impressive and I later discovered it was the first school for the deaf in Britain, which also used a method to develop speech rather than sign language.

Thomas Braidwood was a Scottish mathematics teacher who took on the education of the deaf son of a well-to-do businessman. Soon the boy was able to speak quite well and Braidwood's school in Edinburgh grew. As expected, it was inspected by the ubiquitous Lord Monboddo, who was impressed by the method. The school became so widely known that Dr Johnson and James Boswell also visited Braidwood's school on their famous tour of Scotland. Despite Dr Johnson's famous scepticism they were full of admiration for its results.

Schools for the deaf using Braidwood's oral technique became well established throughout the United Kingdom and the lip-reading skills of the students were noted though they also used signs. Much is made of the "secrecy" around this method and it is sometimes presented in a pejorative manner as though the teachers were trying to protect a monopoly in order to make money. I am sure that it is untrue, even malicious, as the teachers who tried to get their pupils to lip-read and speak were just as dedicated as those who confined themselves to signing. In my opinion they were human, showing pride and jealousy. Each may have claimed special skills and indeed may have had them, much as all professionals hope they have personal qualities to offer. The schools were open to visitors who came frequently but it is true that Thomas Gallaudet had not been well received and that was why he went on to Sicard's school in Paris.

A real criticism of the oral method is that it requires much time and effort which could, in theory, be put to better use in acquiring general learning rather than barely intelligible speech. This criticism is still justified if little progress is made with speech, which probably depends more on how profound the deafness is and how early it was acquired than on the intelligence and perseverance of both pupil and teacher.

The invention of electricity and of the amplifier gave an extraordinary boost to the oral schools and another family quickly took centre stage this time.

Another Scot, a shoemaker called Alexander Bell, decided to leave his trade to study elocution and become an actor at the Royal Theatre in Edinburgh, where he took part in the famous play *l'Abbé de l'Épée*. The play had done extremely well in Paris and now played to packed houses all over Europe. Alexander also began giving lessons to people with speech problems, and when his wife left him for another man, he moved to London with his sons to begin a career teaching and writing on speech defects. One of his son, Melville, eventually returned to Edinburgh where he became a lecturer in elocution and married a woman who was herself deaf, though with some residual hearing. With Melville's help she was eventually able to play and teach the piano by placing an ear trumpet against the instrument. Melville became interested in phonetics and George Bernard Shaw even referred to his work in the preface to his play *Pygmalion*. It was Melville's techniques that were used by Professor Higgins in the play, as well as the musical adaptation, *My Fair Lady*.

Melville's son, Alexander Graham Bell, was invited to America to teach elocution. While he was there he took courses in electricity and mechanics at the new Massachusetts Institute of Technology. He gave lectures at Harvard and taught at the new Boston University, becoming prominent in the intellectual life of Boston. He married Mabel Hubbard, a profoundly deaf woman who had been born hearing and was anxious to maintain her speech and to integrate into hearing society. This led him to try to make an electric amplifier before going on to invent the telephone and many other appliances.

Amplification and the development of the hearing aid meant that numerous children who only had a partial hearing loss could be taught and encouraged to hear enough to learn good speech; concurrently, lip-reading skills became much easier to acquire.

On a final note on educating the deaf, the 1952 film *Mandy* tells the story of a deaf girl whose dedicated mother would not take no for an answer. She brought her child to a school where the girl was taught to speak by the headmaster, played by Jack Hawkins. The film was so emotionally charged that it had a considerable influence on public perception of deaf education. The Ewings' school in Manchester was used as a model both for the film and for the training of teachers.

8.2 Deaf Children Today

8.2.1 *Screening*

It is the screening process that has failed if a deaf child has not been identified until it is obvious that speech failed to develop.

Congenital deafness is often associated with other abnormalities and complete medical assessment of the whole child as well as of the hearing loss is the first step, but not every single hospital can offer every type of service, as a paediatric audiology centre is a highly specialised enterprise.

8.2.2 *Fitting hearing aids*

Now that we have tiny but powerful hearing aids it is possible to fit even very young children. This is not without problems as they have to fit exactly and this requires making plastic ear moulds of the size of the ear canal. As the baby grows so quickly they have to be refitted frequently. Hearing aids are described in more detail in Section 8.3.

8.2.3 *Early training*

Training should start as soon as the diagnosis is made, even if the child is only six months old. Yet general education at school only starts at the age of five, a gap too great to be acceptable in the case of deaf children. In the United Kingdom and many other countries the response has been the establishment of a very good system of peripatetic teachers who are based in the units where the assessments are made.

The term "peripatetic" assures that the teacher has the authority to go from place to place, see the deaf child at home, in the clinic or in a nursery where it might be placed. The system has proved a successful way of helping small children in their own environment. The focus is less on lessons to the child but on teaching the mother and other close members of the family ways to help the child and how to handle the hearing aid. Visits include answering questions from family or nursery attendants, and the teachers act as a contact with the clinic and education authorities. Unfortunately, the effectiveness of the system is too often blighted by shortages of staff.

8.2.4 *Education*

The social outlook of the past few decades has involved a widespread desire to integrate everything and everybody. Indeed, the school system as a whole is now called "Comprehensive" and this inclusiveness, emotional as well as political, takes in those children with disabilities as well. However, we are now witnessing debates on "specialist" schools and "faith" schools and it may well be that, as a society, we are in the process of changing our minds yet again, so that integration may cease to be the main objective. How this will affect the education of deaf children is still not clear but we must use the changing outlook to obtain even better facilities and specialised equipment for our deaf children.

8.2.5 *Mainstream schools*

If the child has developed speech by the age of five he may be able enter the mainstream school system especially if it is in a small class. The teacher may wear a radio transmitter round her neck while the child has receiver hearing aids so that the teacher's words will not be affected by the noise of the class.

In ideal circumstances the child will make good progress and be able to keep up with the class. A peripatetic teacher may come in frequently, both to give him extra tuition in areas where he is not at his best and also to help his class teacher to understand the hearing aid and techniques useful in teaching the deaf.

The class may be large, however, and the staff harassed, while the local authority may be unable to provide specialist help. The burden then falls on the parents who have to know what the child needs to do in class and try not to let it fall behind. When this goes beyond the parents' skills and knowledge, they may be able to get extra help from a private teacher, although this may sometimes not be possible for financial reasons, or be offensive, in principle, to those who refuse to countenance anything outside state provision.

I have occasionally come across unhelpful or insecure teachers who feel unable to handle the presence of a child with a hearing loss and who wears hearing aids in their class.

8.2.6 *Special units*

Some schools have special units for their deaf children. Many are well staffed and have good equipment and are suitable if the child is unable to cope in an ordinary class but has adequate speech. These units can provide the special teaching needed and the electronic technology available.

They have the advantage of access to the other facilities offered by the school and, of course, contact with other children.

8.2.7 *Special schools*

There are a number of schools for deaf children that have a very fine tradition and produce remarkable results with very profoundly deaf children.

It is here that the question of manual communication looms largest, and where the demands for the abandonment of precious teaching time in order to produce only inadequate speech have been greatest.

Signing systems have been discussed already, and there has also been great interest in mouth–hand systems; in other words, oral communication with a manual supplement. The most popular is called "cued speech" and was invented by Dr Orin Cornett at Gallaudet University to help with the comprehension of phonemes that cannot be distinguished from each other by looking at the lips alone, such as /p/ and /b/. Lip-reading or speech reading, as it is often called, uses the lips for as much information as they can give, but there are aspects of speech such as rhythm, intonation and inflection which are closely related to the syllables and cannot be deduced from reading lips.

Cued speech follows the syllables by placing the fingers near the mouth to give "cues" which supplement the lip movements. There are a number of advantages to this method as it enhances normal lip-reading by drawing attention to the mouth, and it supplements rather than detracts from any residual hearing. As it signifies the syllables it follows the rhythm of speech and it is not too difficult for the average family to learn.

In 1880 a world congress held in Milan came to the conclusion that deaf children should be taught to lip-read and speak as best they can as that was the way to give them the best chance in a hearing society. Ever since then oralism became the standard of deaf education.

Nevertheless a proportion of children were unable to acquire adequate speech and gravitated towards using sign language among themselves. Initially they were considered "failures" except among the followers of Gallaudet and a few other establishments, but in the 1960s sign language began to establish itself as a language in its own right.

This was accompanied by the realisation that the academic attainment of deaf children as a whole was unacceptably low and it was the "oral failures" themselves who led a revolt against the imposition of speech by hearing teachers. There was much bitterness in their assertion that these teachers' obsession with oral communication had deprived many of them of the real education to which they had been entitled.

Few people were prepared to refute their arguments even though they were often couched in the aggressive terms common in the 1960s and 1970s. These were similar to the statements of others who considered themselves deprived minorities and, not infrequently, seemed designed to accuse and provoke rather than to persuade.

The facts however were there. Deaf children were not, as a group, doing as well as they should in education, while institutions such as Gallaudet University, committed to sign language, were going from strength to strength.

Reversing the policy of oralism, dominant for almost 100 years, was difficult however, not least because the vast majority of teachers were not deaf themselves and had little knowledge of sign language.

Nevertheless a growing tendency towards signing led many people to wonder why the deaf should not make use of whatever means were at their disposal, oral or manual, and the outcome became known as total communication or TC. Despite some rather entrenched views among the oralists and the manualists, many teachers use TC where it seems particularly useful, especially with infants and very young children when a valid assessment of the degree of hearing loss and suitability of hearing aids is not possible.

In summary, the speech that we can expect from a deaf child depends on the age when the hearing was lost, when it was first discovered, the use of electrical aids to hearing, including cochlear implants, and the provision of training programmes, as well as on how profound the deafness is.

There are many other factors. Some relate to the child, such as intelligence, personality and the presence or absence of other abnormalities. A great deal also depends on the family and health, persistence and personality of the mother. The social conditions of the home also add to their ability to help the child and to make the most of the guidance given.

8.3 Hearing Aids

In 1948 it was agreed that hearing aids, together with glasses, false teeth and, unexpectedly, wigs, were to be provided free of charge to whoever needed them. What was not specified was which particular ones, though "cosmetic" considerations were excluded as that was a concept not favoured in those postwar egalitarian times.

As different types of aid continue to be offered, an ongoing dialogue has taken place between the consumer and the producer as to what is the "best" or "most suitable" as the two are not quite the same, a discussion complicated by the presence of a third party that is supposed to bear the cost, the state.

For the administration, the best hearing aid is undeniably the cheapest. For the specialist, the best is the one which provides the clearest speech discrimination. Many consumers however, would choose the one which is the least visible even if the quality were not as good or the cost out of proportion though this is rarely expressed openly.

On the other hand a very narrow canal may simply not admit a particular coveted aid and older people with arthritic fingers and poor vision should be cautious before paying a great deal of money for the smallest aids with even tinier batteries which they may never be able to handle or even see properly.

The process of choosing a hearing aid therefore involves three separate aspects: the cost, the quality of hearing that it provides and the appearance that we find most acceptable. Inevitably compromises have to be made.

An ideal procedure would be to see a doctor, preferably a specialist, who will check that there is no serious disease involved. The degree and nature of the hearing loss is usually assessed by pure tone audiometry and the aid itself issued or sold by an NHS or independent audiologist. As it has been estimated that 85% of the hearing loss in the population is now age-related and there is little doubt that the demand will increase very rapidly, it may not be possible to offer examination by a specialist in every case. Trained audiologists will have to detect those patients who should be investigated further and it is to them that we turn to service, clean and repair the aid.

8.3.1 *Amplifying sound*

No doubt the first attempt at aiding the hearing must have been to hold the hand cupped behind the ear so as to collect the sound and direct it towards the ear canal. This simple method increases the sound by about 5 dB and also encourages people to raise their voices.

Anything that can collect sound in this way is helpful and it is said that the feathered headdresses worn by American Indians served this purpose. Sea shells and animal horns also offer this degree of amplification and implements of a similar shape were fashioned in different materials and built into fans, umbrellas and even women's hats. Speaking into a rolled newspaper pointed at a person's ear also produces considerable amplification. René Laennec, the French physician who has a hospital in Paris named after him, is said to have designed the first stethoscope based on that principle. It was from manufacturers of such devices that in the 1880s attempts to use electricity to amplify sounds emerged although the first electrical hearing aids developed out of the telephone.

Its inventor was Alexander Graham Bell (see Section 8.1.3) and his hearing aids were initially called "carbon type" because they contained two pieces of carbon through which a current was passed. The resistance to its passage depended on how closely the carbons were pressed together as the tighter they were, the easier it was for the current to flow between them.

One of the carbon pieces was fixed and the other free, attached only to a thin diaphragm with which it vibrated in response to sound so that the resulting slight changes in the distance between them altered the resistance in the current in time with the vibrations turning it into a simple microphone. To amplify the power of the current which had been generated by a battery, a vacuum tube was introduced like the valves of the old radios. The current then came to a receiver, a reverse arrangement from the microphone, which converted it back into sound vibrations. Since its power had been much increased, the sound was now louder than the original one.

I cannot quite understand why it took so long to invent both the telephone and the hearing aid. People were fascinated by science in the 18th century and public lectures were attended by large numbers of both men and women all over Europe and America. Demonstrations were often held showing the transformation of sound into electricity and electromagnetic changes were also converted into sound by inducing the vibration of a diaphragm. It was well known too that electricity could pass along an insulated wire and yet no telephone was made until 1876.

All the necessary knowledge to make one was available since 1836, just about the time that Queen Victoria came to the throne. Probably what was lacking was not the science but the entrepreneurial skills of Alexander Graham Bell, and had Bell's own wife not been deaf he may not have tried to make a hearing aid. Even then, this did not appear until 1900. As it was, he encountered considerable hostility from those who favoured sign language as a means of expression as soon as he began to use amplification in teaching the congenitally deaf to speak. Bell's entrepreneurial prowess also irritated academic scientists when it led to a commercially viable telephone and to the Bell Telephone Company.

The original hearing aid, with its battery and vacuum tube amplifier, must have been very unwieldy. Indeed, we have had to wait until the transistor, the integrated circuit and the computer were invented before it could be miniaturised.

The basic system which forms a hearing aid even now is relatively simple. It starts with a microphone which turns sound vibrations of the diaphragm into the fluctuations of an electrical signal. An amplifier then increases the strength of the signal using power from a battery and it finally reaches the earphone, an electromagnetic device which sets up vibrations in another diaphragm. As the current is now stronger the sound is louder.

If the microphone is held too near the earphone a phenomenon called *feedback* occurs, a sort of self-amplification, so that the whole system emits a high pitched whistling sound which the deaf person may not be able to hear but which is very disturbing to others in the vicinity. This can also happen if the device is too near a reflecting surface such as a wall.

Feedback was not a problem, even when the volume was turned right up, when the aid was a box pinned to the clothing on the chest, well away from the earphone, but when miniaturisation came and everything was fitted into a small apparatus worn behind the ear the only way to prevent it was for a perfectly fitting ear mould closing off the canal so that no acoustic leakage would occur.

The mould is made from an impression of the canal taken by a self-curing silicone which is then reproduced in acrylic, vinyl or other substance.

8.3.2 *Expectations*

As in all things expectations must be realistic if we are to avoid frustration and dissatisfaction.

If the hearing has diminished to the point where it is not possible to converse without embarrassment, where this interferes with social life, listening to sermons in church or attending lectures; if the radio or television requires a volume that offends others, then a hearing aid would be very helpful. It might also help to mask irritating tinnitus by bringing in environmental sounds.

On the other hand a hearing aid cannot replace normal hearing. It presents difficulties in background noise such as restaurants, particularly those with reflecting surfaces to increase a "buzzing" atmosphere. A hearing aid is not much help at a cocktail party.

Problems are countless and however many we try to address in advance there will always be an unexpected one so there is no alternative to a good relationship with the hearing aid dispenser. Many of the problems are related to the nature of the deafness. If there is no hearing in the higher frequencies then no amount of amplification will conjure up the sounds and "*sss*" or "*fff*" will simply not be heard whatever the quality of the hearing aid.

Some types of deafness involve a very narrow dynamic range which means that there is not much distance between sounds being too loud and not loud enough.

Some people are allergic to the plastic material of the ear mould and this may cause eczema and, at times when it gets infected, otitis externa.

There are various different materials available and on one occasion I had even arranged to have the mould gold-plated to avoid sensitivity because gold is so inert. Bone conductor hearing aids are also often used in these cases and occasionally bone anchored hearing aids (see Section 8.3.4.9).

8.3.3 *Two hearing aids*

It is much better to have an aid in each ear rather than just in one ear (provided the hearing loss is bilateral, of course). Less power is used and the volume does not have to be turned on as high and it is more effective in background noise.

Most valuable is the stereophonic impact which gives better perception of space and depth so that it is possible to localise where sounds are coming from, and there is also the social benefit of not being forced to ignore the person on the "deaf side".

8.3.4 *Hearing aid types*

Body worn hearing aids, which are pinned to the clothing with a wire running to the earphone, are now rarely prescribed except for very small children. The majority of hearing aids can be divided into those worn behind the ear, in the ear, in the canal and the very small ones which disappear entirely inside the canal.

8.3.4.1 *Behind the ear*

These are larger than the others but offer a number of advantages. As they are bigger, there is room for more powerful amplifiers and larger batteries that last longer. The case which fits behind the ear can be matched with the skin for colour. The sound is directed by a transparent plastic tube and mould into the canal. Another advantage of size is that the parts are easier to see and handle.

There are mini behind-the-ear types with a very slim casing that fits under the hair line and a clear plastic tube or even a fine wire to a receiver embedded in the ear mould. These are known as receiver in the canal or

RIC aids and have more advantages as they require less power and are therefore more efficient. There is less feedback so the volume can be increased for the more severely deaf. The speaker or receiver is in the canal so it does not have to occlude it and is more comfortable to wear, indeed it can be vented to allow any natural sounds that the listener can still hear to reach the eardrum.

8.3.4.2 *In the ear (ITE) aids*

The advantage of ITE aids over the behind the-ear-aids is that the microphones are in the same position as the normal ear canal so that sound comes in from the right direction. This helps to localise where a sound is coming from. The aid is still large enough to be handled easily.

They work well in mild to moderate hearing loss.

8.3.4.3 *In the canal (ITC) aids*

These go into the canal and are hardly visible but because of their small size cannot be very powerful and are useful only in mild to moderate hearing losses.

8.3.4.4 *Completely in the canal (CTC) aids*

They are so small that they fit entirely within the canal and have to be pulled out by a thin twig but as they are not very powerful they can only be useful to those who have only mild hearing losses. The canal itself has to be wide enough to accept it and, as the battery is so tiny, good vision and adequate manual dexterity is necessary too.

8.3.4.5 *Analogue and digital*

When sound is processed in an analogue manner the sound vibrations have been transformed into a single electric current despite all the complexity of its form. This was how LP recordings were made and how, until very recently, radio and television was transmitted.

Digital processing is quite different as the sound is transformed into digits, 0 and 1 or plus and minus, yes and no or on and off, which makes it possible to manipulate it like a computer, giving it the characteristics that we wish before converting it back into an analogue acoustic signal that we can hear. The processing involves dividing the signal into tiny segments whose pitch and loudness can be measured at every given moment and altered as required.

CDs and DVDs are made that way and transmission of both radio and television will shortly be entirely digital. This technology is already available to hearing aids in miniaturised form and provides better sound quality.

8.3.4.6 Letting in the air

Vents have been made in the moulds of many aids so as to give the ears an "unplugged" feeling by allowing the air into the canal and the natural sound at those frequencies that can be heard without amplification to enter the ear as normal. The problem has been to establish stabilising techniques which prevent the feedback and whistling that an acoustic leak would produce. The combination of digital amplification with normal hearing for those pitches that can be heard gives a much more natural sound.

8.3.4.7 Different programmes

Some hearing aids have the possibility of switching to different processing programmes according to whether the wearer is in a noisy environment or in a quiet situation and some can do this by remote control from a device kept in the pocket.

8.3.4.8 Bone conductor aids

These are necessary if for one reason or another, for example a narrow canal, a chronically discharging ear or a congenital abnormality, it is not possible to fit any sort of aid into the canal.

The principle is simple as a vibrator replaces the receiver of a hearing aid and if pressed on to the bone behind the ear it will transmit sound to the skull and hence directly to the inner ear.

It does not work very well if the hearing loss is neurosensory and it has to be pressed so tightly behind the ear that it is often quite unpleasant. Cosmetically too it is not so easily acceptable as it has to be held in place by a spring around the head like a head-band. The hearing aid can also be placed in the arm of a pair of heavy glasses but this is not as effective.

Altogether I have only found a bone conductor aid helpful in patients with conductive hearing loss.

8.3.4.9 *Bone anchored hearing aids (Baha®)*

This originated in a technique for implanting artificial teeth which are attached to screws made of titanium. This material is strong and light, and so well tolerated by the body's tissues, especially bone, that the living cells actually grow into the pores in the metal.

In Baha® such a screw goes through the skin behind the ear and into the skull. A hearing aid can then be attached to it so that the amplified sound vibrations are transmitted through the bone to the inner ear. It is therefore a bone conductor of sorts and works best with conductive deafness.

It is not without problems as it requires an extensive operation to place it, with all the usual risks of infection that go with any operation. The hearing aid itself is about the size of a matchbox and is naturally intrusive. Moreover, some find the idea of a screw in their head psychologically disturbing.

8.3.4.10 *CROS and BiCROS*

Most people who are completely deaf in one ear only but can hear well in the other usually manage perfectly well without a hearing aid at all, but on occasion they have a problem. Sitting at a noisy dinner table, for instance, they will not be able to hear what someone is saying on their deaf side, and there are obvious professional difficulties for those who have to attend meetings.

One solution, called CROS, involves a pair of glasses with a microphone on the deaf side and the earphone in the hearing ear so that it receives sound from both sides. If that side is also not good a BiCROS aid can be used.

8.3.4.11 *Radio aids*

These are particularly useful in schools where a teacher can wear a transmitter round her neck and the deaf child will receive the amplified words through a radio transmitter directly into his hearing aid. Such devices are also available for hire in some theatres where the microphone is on the stage.

8.3.4.12 *Loops*

Some halls have a loop around them carrying the electromagnetic impulses of the microphone which can then be picked up directly by a special device in many hearing aids and give a direct sound, clearer than what is picked up from the floor of the hall.

8.4 The Cochlear Implant

"Allo! Allo! Tu m'entends?"

The surgeon in the Paris hospital had picked up a microphone and I could see its wire peeping through the bandages that swathed the head of a young Vietnamese girl as she lay in bed not far from the ward where my little brother was recovering from a mastoid operation.

My mother, encouraging me to become a doctor, had asked the surgeon, Professor Maspetiol, to talk to me and he took me to witness something important that he said I should not forget. That was when he introduced me to the Vietnamese girl who did not speak a word of French but nodded with pleasure every time he spoke into the microphone, her face breaking into broad smiles as she said "Ah! Ah!"

That was in the early 1950s and it was the first cochlear implant.

"She is totally deaf," the surgeon said. "Her ear is dead. Nothing can help her, yet the electric current generated by the microphone every time I speak, is heard!"

It meant little to me but I nodded politely and the Vietnamese girl smiled and said, "Ah!"

After I qualified as a doctor and was training to be a specialist, I had listened to Dr Howard House of Los Angeles, who showed a film at a London conference. His brother Bill had implanted an electric device in the inner ear of a totally deaf girl who could hear something when connected to a microphone. She listened to nursery rhymes and was able to tell which ones they were.

The audience applauded but many criticized him behind his back.

"It is only the rhythm she recognises," some whispered. "'Knock knock, knock knock,' is obviously 'Twinkle, Twinkle' and not 'Mary had a Little Lamb'."

It seemed to me that even that was an advantage and as Dr House had not mentioned it had already been done in France, I went up to tell him about the Vietnamese girl in Paris hoping, perhaps, to attract the attention of such a famous American surgeon. He said a reference would be made, in due course, about what he called French experiments.

Later when I had my own unit at Guy's Hospital, the Department of Health invited me to introduce this type of work in the United Kingdom, but first I had to find out exactly what can be heard when an electrical impulse stimulated a dead inner ear. What it sounded like seemed to me the basis of implantation and I had the right patient to help me.

He heard normally in one ear. The other ear, which was a totally deaf, dead ear, had had extensive surgery for life-threatening infection and it had left him with no drum or middle ear and when I looked I could see right down to the bulge of the cochlea itself so it was easy to apply an electrode to its surface.

Fascinated by the project, my patient, who was an intelligent man, was able to compare the sound tones in his good ear with what he heard through electrical stimulation in the other.

As different pitches are the result of vibrations of different frequencies recorded as cycles per second or Hertz, each vibration was transformed into an electrical impulses of the same frequency.

Middle C, a pitch of 250 Hz per second was replaced in the deaf ear by 250 electrical pulses per second and the patient could then tell us if the sound he heard from electrical stimulation at this rate of impulses compared reasonably well with the real sound presented in his good ear.

At the lowest frequencies a modest current sounds similar to the equivalent pitch. As we get to the higher pitches, the strength of the current needed to hear increases, becoming less tolerable and even painful so that our patient could not hear any but the lowest pitches without discomfort.

When I suggested that electrical stimulation could help totally deaf people to understand speech a little better than lip-reading alone, the scientists of a Medical Research Council committee were sceptical but they put me in touch with Dr Adrian Fourcin, an expert in speech.

Dr Fourcin told me that the frequencies that could be heard from electrical stimulation happened also to be those of the voice but that speech itself included a large number of higher pitches such as the sounds "s" and "f" and, indeed, most of the consonants which were not made simply by the voice.

This meant that, at the very least, a cochlear implant could help a deaf person to lip-read as, for instance, we cannot tell the difference between "zoo" and the girl's name "Sue" by only looking at the lips. "I am looking for Sue" looks very much like "I am going to the zoo".

The confusion rests mainly on not being able to tell the difference between the "sss" sound and the "zzz" as the lip movements are the same. The first, however, is "unvoiced" while the second is "voiced". Indeed, we can actually *feel* the difference simply by placing our fingers lightly on the throat. When we say "sss" we feel nothing, when we say "zzz" we can feel the rumble and that difference can be "heard" with electrical stimulation.

We were soon joined by Viennese and Australian groups, and I was anxious to see what was going on in Paris where they were now well advanced. Research and development had continued uninterrupted from the time when the first electrode had been implanted in the Vietnamese girl only a few years after the end of the Second World War.

The Australians were the most successful in making a marketable implantable device with considerable help and encouragement from their government. Indeed, stamps were printed honouring the Bionic Ear.

Few things in the management of deafness have led to more misconceptions than the cochlear implant as it has only limited use, but where it does help it can make an enormous difference to a person's life.

The two main misconceptions are that it can restore the hearing completely and that as it is "implanted" it is all beneath the skin and therefore invisible.

8.4.1 *The apparatus*

The implanted part of the apparatus consists, first of all, of a receiver that is placed beneath the skin behind the ear. It receives electrical impulses across the skin from the outside part of the apparatus and decodes them transmitting the resulting signals along the appropriate electrodes to the inner ear.

Different prostheses have a different number of electrodes and this array is inserted into the cochlea, threaded quite far down along its coiled interior.

When activated, these electrodes will stimulate the parts of the cochlea to which they are closest. In the diseased or damaged organ many sections do not respond at all and have lost their nerve supply. That sets major limits to what can be achieved but the surviving nerve fibres transmit the electrical impulses to the brain.

The external device has a microphone which transforms sound into an electrical wave form which transmits to a computer called a speech processor which picks out the speech patterns and separates out the signals destined for the different electrodes which will enter the cochlea.

This very complex collection of signals is transmitted to the implanted receiver through a coil held in the right place by a magnet.

8.4.2 *What is heard?*

This corresponds to the lower pitches and includes the voice, though not speech as a whole. Lip-reading still has a major place as do other visual signs such as facial expression, but training is so important that it is not worth implanting anyone unless they have the possibility and the willingness to pursue both a pre- and post-operative programme.

The results we can expect depend on selecting those we can help.

8.4.3 *Who can be helped?*

A person who has lost all his or her hearing after having developed speech is the best candidate, the younger the better. The best results are obtained if the hearing has not been lost too long before an implant is considered.

Adults who have been deaf from birth and are unable to speak are the ones least likely to receive much benefit. Those who have been implanted have said that it has helped them in the sense that they became aware of the presence of sound. In itself this is of some value, for instance in being able to hear a door bell, the ringing of a telephone or someone who is trying to attract their attention. On the other hand they can rarely understand speech and learn to speak.

Children are in a different category because if they are born totally deaf they are unlikely to develop speech unless they are implanted early, before the brain has lost its power to learn to process speech.

A cochlear implant is not an option for those people, whether children or adults, who have enough hearing to be able to use a hearing aid.

Chapter 9

When the Hearing is Normal

The problems may be of speech, of language and of brain function.

9.1 Language Deprivation

It is not enough just to be able to hear as it is speech we have to hear before we can learn to speak.

The Borough of Southwark was a deprived district when I started my Hearing and Language Clinic at Guy's Hospital, and many of its families seemed to live isolated from one another. It was quite different in neighbouring borough Bermondsey, and the contrast was then so tangible that residents there were offended when they were mistaken as coming from "the Borough". The problems had started with the destruction of whole streets during the bombing of London in the Second World War, and the subsequent decision to relocate some of the inhabitants in new towns in what was thought to be more salubrious surroundings outside the city. As a result of that policy the population of Southwark had been moved away, and the intention was, in due course to redevelop that area.

That did not happen for decades, and when these ambitious and misguided projects gradually petered out, new migrants began to occupy the dilapidated houses which the authorities had condemned, but not destroyed. They came in dribs and drabs from all over the country and abroad looking for work and many were lonely people who formed lose associations rather than families. Single women were left with small children and no support from nearby friends and relatives, so the number of cases of clinical depression and its complications were high, while young men, drawn by the jobs available in the capital, had sometimes left families behind and relationships were lost. The worst aspect was lack of contact and even hostility from the neighbours.

The saddest comment I remember was from a patient who said they had been burgled and had lost their only possessions, the television and music player. I wondered who could want to rob such impoverished people, but she knew it was the neighbours. She had said angrily that they waited for them to go out to break the door and steal their things.

They brought their children to see us only if the "social" forced them to come. This was clearly a difference with Bermondsey as the people from that borough, although poor, had hung on to their homes for generations. They readily came for their appointments with a mother, a sister, or an old school friend and their children's speech was the lively dialect of south London.

When groups of foreign immigrants came, problems with speech development increased, and many believed that the cause was confusion between the two languages. They were told by well-meaning people that they should speak to their child only in English.

I tried to help a family of Sicilian immigrants as I could speak Italian, although theirs was a rather rough dialect. They had two school-age children who were placed in school immediately but appeared to be in disarray as they had no English. I assured the parents that at least the new baby, born here, would give them no problem.

What did bring them back eventually, though, was not the older children about whom I had been anxious. They now spoke good English and acted as interpreters for the parents. However, the baby was causing the problems: the child was then almost four and hardly spoke at all. His hearing was normal and he was not delayed in any other way, so suspicion fell on the possible confusion of trying to learn two languages at once.

This led to a project aimed at comparing the exposure to two languages. We divided each day of a typical week into three periods of morning, afternoon and evening and we charted the time that English was spoken as well as the time the child was exposed to another language spoken at home.

To my surprise I found that children from bilingual families, who had delayed speech produced blank charts as no one spoke to them at all in

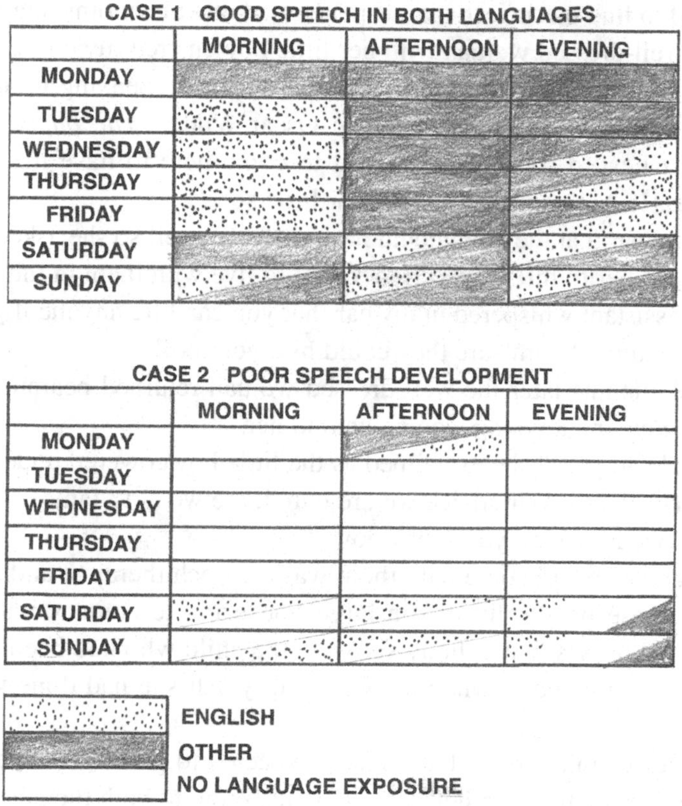

CASE 1 GOOD SPEECH IN BOTH LANGUAGES

	MORNING	AFTERNOON	EVENING
MONDAY			
TUESDAY			
WEDNESDAY			
THURSDAY			
FRIDAY			
SATURDAY			
SUNDAY			

CASE 2 POOR SPEECH DEVELOPMENT

	MORNING	AFTERNOON	EVENING
MONDAY			
TUESDAY			
WEDNESDAY			
THURSDAY			
FRIDAY			
SATURDAY			
SUNDAY			

ENGLISH

OTHER

NO LANGUAGE EXPOSURE

Figure 23. Deprivation.

any language (Figure 22). The Sicilian family confessed that the little boy was taken to a child minder in the morning and picked up when the parents had finished work. He was then fed, and quickly put to bed so that the other children could do their homework.

We visited a number of child minders and although some of them were good, others took in too many children who were placed in cots with the curtains drawn in the hope that they might go to sleep, so the problem was not one of confusion of languages but of lack of exposure to any at all.

As speech deprivation also means a degree of social deprivation, it was often associated with inadequate home conditions. Our work helped establish the registration and inspection of child minders but I was surprised to find our investigations penetrated other economic classes too, when a well-dressed woman with her little boy entered my clinic without an appointment and addressed us in superior tones speaking in the same manner I imagine Lady Bracknell in Oscar Wilde's *The Importance of Being Earnest* to speak: "I was told to come here to have his hearing checked. He can't speak a word, poor little sod!"

It was clear that the child could hear perfectly well so she asked loudly if I advised her to hire a speech therapist to live with them in the country and my assistant whispered in my ear that you can hire anyone if you pay enough, adding, "I am sure they could hire you too!"

A few months later the well-dressed woman returned beaming, dragging the boy and a young woman behind her.

"Thanks to you!" she exclaimed as the little boy cowered underneath a table. "Thanks to your advice we are cured, are we not? James, show the good doctor how well you speak now!"

The girl who had come with them was a speech therapist and she told me that these people lived in a large house in the country with dogs, stables and horses, but nobody spoke to the child who had been running wild, and just came in when he was hungry. All she had done was talk to him.

Another couple, young but already expected to go far, as indeed they have done since they are both now famous, brought both their little sons, one almost three and the other around four, to see me as neither of them spoke.

Though the mother was somewhat distant, the father was engaging and friendly. As both parents worked, I asked who looked after the children. They insisted that there was no problem at all, as they had an arrangement with a Scandinavian nanny agency that was completely in charge and, if the nanny was ill or unhappy, all she has to do was to call for a replacement who would be sent at once. The father looked thoughtful and added:

"Do you think that perhaps they can speak Swedish?" nodding towards the boys.

No class, culture or social group is entirely free from elements of deprivation, and where there is language deprivation it is difficult to avoid emotional deprivation too.

9.2 Mental Disability

Though we have known since the time of Broca that certain parts of the brain are associated with language (see Section 5.7), it was only when we became familiar with computers that we began to use new words like "processing", both to hide our ignorance of what is really going on in the brain and to indicate that we have, at last, a clue. When the electrical impulses that represent words reach the brain they are "processed" and it is from that activity, whatever it may be, that language results. It is where our perceptual, cognitive, motor and social abilities reside and where our semantic and syntactic skills are expressed, and there is a close correlation between language development and intellectual growth.

Brain function could be impaired as a result of a congenital abnormality, by damage from infection such as in meningitis, or by injury, which includes birth trauma and where resulting learning difficulties may be only part of a global delay. There is sometimes motor delay as well, for instance, with the child unable to walk or feed himself so that language failure does not stand out as a single problem. The scale of the delay and what it implies can often be gauged by the early milestones in the child's development.

Language performs an important function in regulating all human activity so that the development of social maturation and therefore behaviour, cognitive abilities and emotional stability will be related to success in achieving language and if the child is severely disabled, he may fail to develop language altogether. If the disability is less severe he may have the basic processes which initiate the development of language but may never do this fully or at least be delayed.

Symbolic play is an important guide to the degree of delay, and observing how a child plays with toys such as a little table with its chairs, cups and saucers, and dolls allows us to see how even the two year old understands that the toys are symbols for the real ones and will go through the motions of pouring imaginary tea and offering the tiny cup to the dolls. If the child can do this, verbal instructions can be given which become more and more complex to assess the degree of understanding.

Those who do the assessing have to be highly skilled as there are very frequently more than one problem and they are difficult to disentangle.

A child with a learning disability may also have a hearing loss, and failure to respond to instructions may be due to that.

In general, with intellectual disability, everything is delayed, words come late and are acquired only slowly, and phrases and sentences appear later than they should. There are often other problems of maturity, such as difficulty with attention, and with listening, while the child is easily distracted and often hyperactive. Sometimes there are major behavioural abnormalities such as rocking or head banging.

9.3 Specific Language Disorders

The term "language delay" at first means what it says: that language has not yet appeared and but it is transient. "Language disorder" implies a permanent problem and should be used only later, when other causes of delay, such as hearing loss or deprivation have been excluded or dealt with.

During the 1960s, among the children we saw who suffered from impaired intellectual development a group was described as showing particular features. They seemed to be unable to perceive other peoples' emotions and although there was clearly a cognitive defect which reduced their ability to reason, the difficulty they had with communication tended to dominate their disorder. Unlike some other forms of intellectual retardation, these children showed that their communication problem affected non-linguistic as well as linguistic capabilities as it involved gesture, touch, facial expression, eye contact and gaze as well as speech.

It was in this way that we were introduced to the term "autism" and, as it was presented as a new discovery rather than as a shift in terminology there was great excitement. There was hope also, as a new disease may mean new treatment and the chance of progress. This classification was difficult to use as children rarely fall into carefully defined groups, and so we started using the term "autistic features" when describing those who suffered particularly from non-linguistic communication problems such as refusal to seek eye contact as well as linguistic ones.

In time we found that a high percentage had learning difficulties which we began to call "learning disorder with autistic features", and since then the diagnosis has broadened so much that autism seems to encompass almost the whole range of learning disorders and children often appear to be placed somewhere along an "autistic spectrum".

9.3.1 *Specific language impairment*

If the hearing is not impaired and intellectual development is adequate, and there is no likelihood of emotional or linguistic deprivation nor are there obvious psychological problems, and yet the child has failed to speak, then there is a problem of what to call the condition, particularly as the diagnosis is only arrived at by excluding other ones.

The term "developmental aphasia" was in use for a while although it carried neurological implications which were better understood in elderly patients with strokes.

We then talked of specific language disorder (SLD) and now of specific language impairment (SLI) which are helpful terms to describe children who have not developed language adequately but are otherwise normal, though it would be wrong to make such a diagnosis until the age of four years old.

Withholding a diagnosis in the hope that as maturation progresses the problem will disappear spontaneously is the right thing to do as this happens in so many children. On the other hand it is hardly possible to do so without giving some sort of reassurance simply in order to survive while waiting, though this often angers the parents if the expected progress does not take place. It leaves them with the feeling that the doctor had missed the diagnosis or that their anxieties had been wantonly disregarded. Either way it does not help the parents but I have found over the years that honesty remains the best course though this does not mean bluntness and certainly not brutality.

Most parents will understand that it is not a matter of diagnosing a disease but of questioning the way development occurs, so that there is no alternative to watching how things unfold.

As usual, the developmental failures produce quite a broad spectrum of problems of varying degrees of severity, though attempts have been made to separate those which are entirely or mainly to do with expression only, from those which also involve comprehension.

Some have phonological problems, which means that the difficulty lies in perceiving and producing sounds. It may present simply as immature speech which persists longer than about the age of three. To delete the final consonant such as when saying *"ba'"* instead of "ball" and *"ha'"* instead of "hat" may be normal in the young child but after the age of three should give some cause for concern. They may also present in a manner deviant from the normal as well as delayed in maturity in which case it is reasonable to call it a disorder.

Vocabulary may be less extensive than in other children even though it seems more often to be a problem of producing the words than of understanding them but failure to put words together by the age of two is an indication that there may be delay.

Children with SLI seem to be more likely to suffer from other problems such as poor attention, clumsiness, poor eye–finger coordination, and slowness in absorbing auditory information. We should be aware of this when working out methods for helping these children as a slower, more patient, input from the teacher makes a considerable difference. Other signs such as clumsiness should also be taken into consideration and helped.

The term *dyspraxia* is used when there are problems in articulating even though the muscles used for speech are normal. They function quite normally in smiling, licking, sucking and involuntary movements and it is only speaking that they cannot do.

Sometimes we find syntactic disorders where grammar is abnormal and articles, pronouns, prepositions and suffixes disappear. In the more serious cases, the disorder also shows semantic difficulties, as the meaning of words is affected.

Parents of children with language delay often report social and behavioural problems including lack of attention, hyperactivity, moodiness and even aggression though, in my experience, these tend to resolve as the language difficulties improve.

The cause of language disorder or impairment, like that of autism remains unknown but there is a definite genetic and hereditary factor as it is four times more common in boys and tends to run in families.

I myself have never been confident that we are dealing with a "disorder" at all. Just as some children are gifted musicians while others are tone deaf; some can draw beautifully while others cannot; some are good at maths while others have enormous trouble with figures, I wonder whether some children are simply bad at language.

As a doctor I have had a problem, however, because language skills are central to our society and no one can do without, and parents therefore ask for their child to be "cured". I could not avoid this request so I had to guide them towards those who could offer the right education with the most appropriate teaching methods.

I have remained an observer, perhaps an unnecessary one as my contribution was so limited, partly out of interest, or even curiosity, but also out of concern and I have tried to obtain some idea as to the prognosis.

On the other hand, I have been an independent witness as I have not been directly responsible for the management or indeed the assessment of these children and my observations must have some value due to their detachment. Not unexpectedly, I have found that when the problem has not been severe the end result has been good. The best guide as to the prognosis has been related to comprehension. If the child's ability to understand is adequate and his difficulties are limited to expression, the ultimate results have been the most satisfactory. All of them responded to intensive special teaching which I felt should not be stinted.

As time went on those children whose difficulties persisted tended to show more specific deficiencies usually related to reading and writing and were labelled *dyslexic*.

9.3.2 *Problems pronouncing*

When a child suffers with difficulties in coordinating the movements of the muscles we use to speak he is often said to suffer from *dysarthria*.

It is of course quite different from *dyspraxia* where the muscles that allow us to form the words can technically function but are unable to do so for the more obscure reasons of inadequate processing.

The symptoms of dysarthria may be mild or severe. Most of the severe cases are children with cerebral palsy, and the spasticity may incapacitate the child badly in other ways. Incoordination of limb movements means that gesture too is limited and there may also be difficulties with feeding and swallowing as well as excessive drooling.

It is quite possible that there may be multiple handicaps such as deafness, visual problems and intellectual deficits and in some cases the child may understand perfectly well and as a result assessments are often very difficult to make.

In the less severe cases the child may have difficulties in moving the tongue, lips and palate so that speech is slurred, laboured, nasal, breathy and not fluent.

9.3.3 *Elective mutism*

Another aspect regarding the inability to speak that must be taken into consideration are the psychological factors.

One little girl was brought to us once; as in many cases she was three years old, the age at which parents begin to worry. The nursery school was concerned and the mother, who seemed to be extremely shy, was not clear as to whether anything was wrong.

The whole episode had been unsatisfactory for them as the two of them, the mother and the little girl, had not been able to push past the more assertive mothers of the Borough of Southwark or their aggressive children and had spent some hours sitting in a distant corner of the clinic not having had the courage to come forward.

We could not come to any conclusion as the child hid her face in her mother's lap and neither said anything nor looked at us but after a few attempts I could see that her speech was definitely immature even for her age and she made only slow progress.

When the time came for her to go to school a year or so later she was referred back to us as now she would not speak at all. She was sensitive and shy but was able to participate in all school activities that did not involve speaking.

She was gradually wooed into speaking very softly provided she too was addressed in a soft voice, and our therapist came to the conclusion that the origins of her mutism was her earlier frustration at not being able to make herself understood. She had not been able to face the resulting social effect nor to make the effort to improve and had simply withdrawn into silence.

I have seen children who would not speak in the clinic or at school but who apparently spoke at home. Very interestingly there were also some who were prepared to speak only to other children.

In my clinic I found that it was mainly girls and their mothers who were shy. Nevertheless there are sometimes very serious causes for elective mutism and these children should be seen by the child psychologist.

9.3.4 *Prevalence of speech and language problems*

There have been many studies of speech and language issues among children in many cities and countries and some have involved thousands of children.

What people take seriously and what they do not varies greatly from place to place and culture to culture but, by and large, it seems that between 5–6% of children still have a speech impairment at the age of five. The vast majority have articulation and expression difficulties rather than those of comprehension; it is more common in boys.

It occurs in children of average, below average and above average intelligence and does not seem to be related to social class. The vast majority are normal in other ways.

The most important aspect is early assessment to exclude hearing loss and to recognise the more serious cases of language disorder. The management is then centred on speech clinics with a spread from supervision and reassurance to more intensive therapy.

Postscript

Melodies Still Unheard

There is an immediacy to hearing as, unlike the eye, the ear cannot scan a scene again and again, checking a thousand times what it perceives. The ear has to decode what it has heard immediately as it deals with something that does not usually repeat itself and people sometimes do not listen and often do not want to hear.

Odysseus in Homer's *The Odyssey* blocked his sailors' ears so that they would not hear the beautiful voices of the Sirens who would lure them to destruction on the rocks. He wanted to make sure that they would also ignore the orders that he himself might give, as he wished to hear the songs of the Sirens. He had himself chained to the mast because he had been warned that, like all men, he would be seduced by the Sirens' song.

In that story, Homer, who is said to have been blind and dependent on his hearing, gives us tantalising clues to the darker consequences of being able to hear. The urge to experience the dangerous, perhaps thrilling, melodies of the Sirens is overwhelming for Odysseus; yet he has been warned that he must be restrained forcefully if he is to listen to the song. The heroes who had listened to the songs had been seduced and were destined to remain on the Sirens' island and rot to death. Posthomeric legend has it that the Sirens themselves would die if someone heard their singing but escaped them. Odysseus and his crew were not, however, the first to escape the Sirens as Orpheus in the *Argonautica*[10]

---

[10] Apollonius Rhodius *Argonautica*: Book IV, line 891.

simply picks up his lyre and drowns them out as he plays even more beautifully than they can sing.

These stories, which connect journeys into temptation and the unknown with hearing and deafness, have been so compelling through the ages that we should not dismiss them out of hand. Each generation can rethink them using its own tools. Franz Kafka wrote in 1917 that although a few people had got away with hearing what the Sirens had to offer, none had escaped their truly fatal weapon: total silence.[11] He implied that what we really apprehend is that we can hear no one speaking to us or that there is, in fact, nothing to say.

Today we often find it easier to understand the world in terms of models, intellectual structures that we can study and continuously modify. Sound can be regarded as making an impression on the mind which responds to fundamental electrical rhythms that can capture the brain in a sort of ultimate melody. Computers are now so much part of our lives that algebraic models best express what happens. Activity occurs within many simple interconnecting units and is called "parallel distributing processing" or "neural networks" according to whether we feel more comfortable with mathematical or biological symbolism (though to me they are synonymous). The units are connected to one another, activation spreading around this network modified by the strengths or weaknesses of the particular connections, the level of activity in a unit depending on what it receives from others as some excite while others inhibit. These models "learn" and can be trained to associate input with output patterns.

Although this approach is being applied to the study of language with some success it still does not help us understand the relationship between language and thought. Did they originate separately or was one driven by the other? They have become interdependent anyway, and I wonder whether the interminable quest for the soul is in fact a search for a unified theory of language, just as the physicists' efforts to understand nature is also sought through a unified theory.

Hector Berlioz had never learned to play an instrument properly other than the drums and he claimed in his memoirs, serialised in the journal *Le Monde Illustré*, that this allowed him to compose freely and in silence,

---

[11] Franz Kafka, *The Silence of the Sirens* (Martin Secker, London: 1933)

delivering him from the tyranny of the fingers "so dangerous to thought, and from the fascination which ordinary sonorities always exercise on a composer."[12] This point of view makes one wonder whether Beethoven's deafness helped to free him from convention allowing his "inner ear" to create radically different compositions.

It may be this inaudible music that Keats refers to in his *Ode to a Grecian Urn*:

> Heard melodies are sweet, but those unheard
> Are sweeter; therefore, ye soft pipes, play on;
> Not to the sensual ear, but, more endear'd
> Pipe to the spirit ditties of no tone.

---

[12] Hector Berlioz, *Memoirs of Hector Berlioz: From 1803 to 1865* (translated by Ernest Newman, Dover Publications, New York: 1966, p. 14).

Further Reading

Further reading is not, of course, compulsory and I trust that this book stands on its own.

Humans used sound initially as a means to warn each other; later it was used to express feeling in music and song. It has been shaped into words and strung together to make grammatical sentences, which could then be ordered into poems that steer the emotions.

The story of how we perceive sound through hearing and how it has helped us teach one another as well as to transmit memories of the past requires more than the consultation of a few volumes so, when I look around my bookshelves, I want to include everything. Should not history itself be covered? Would novels not be appropriate when considering human communication? Should not writing itself be taken into account too, since our alphabets are a symbolic notation of sounds?

Nonetheless, some books have informed me more than others, some are responsible for helping me face the problems of hearing and language in my work and others I have simply found intriguing, so I have listed them here in the hope that they may be useful to others.

Brian C.J. Moore was a friend and a collaborator in my early work on the cochlear implant and I have always felt that his book *Introduction to the Psychology of Hearing* (Academic Press, London: 1977) was written to guide people like me.

Another introduction to phonetics and speech that has remained helpful is Keith Johnson's *Acoustic and Auditory Phonetics* (Basil Blackwell Inc., Oxford: 1997).

I have been much moved as well as informed by Harlan Lane's remarkable history *When the Mind Hears: A History of the Deaf* (Random House, New York: 1984) and I urge those interested in the history and background of the teaching and care of the deaf to read it.

Music has from the start had such a close connection with science and was long considered a branch of mathematics so it is not surprising that it is now inching into scientific works almost as a branch of neuroscience and there are no end of books published that approach it, to some extent, in that way. I have found the following helpful:

Philip Ball, *The Music Instinct: How Music Works and Why We Can't Do Without It* (The Bodley Head, London: 2010).

Jonathan Berger and Gabe Turow, *Music, Science and the Rhythmic Brain: Cultural and Clinical Implications* (Routledge, Abingdon, New York: 2013).

Deryck Cooke, *The Language of Music* (Oxford University Press, Oxford: 1959).

Jean-Jacques Nattiez, *Music and Discourse* (translated by Carolyn Abbate, Princeton University Press, New Jersey: 1990).

Aniruddh D. Patel, *Music, Language, and the Brain* (Oxford University Press, Oxford: 2008).

Charles Rosen, *The Frontiers of Meaning: The Informal Lectures on Music* (Hill & Wang, New York: 1994).

Anthony Storr, *Music and the Mind* (Random House, Inc., New York 1992).

Language has been a real delight and I could never resist elbowing my way into child development and language, which is considered a section of paediatrics. Many thought that area of medicine should be safeguarded from surgeons such as myself but Mary Sheridan, one of the founders of that speciality helped me be a part of it so it is with fond memories that I recommend the edition, updated and revised by Ajay Sharma and Helen Cockerill of Mary Sheridan's *From Birth to Five Years* (Routledge, New York: 2007). Also invaluable is Mathew Saxton's *Child Language: Acquisition and Development* (Sage, London: 2010).

Other books on language which have fascinated me are:

Peter Daniels and William Bright (Eds), *The World's Writing Systems* (Oxford University Press, Oxford: 1996).

W. John Hackwell, *Signs, Letters, Words: Archaeology Discovers Writing* (Scribners, New York: 1987).

Nigel Lewis, *The Book of Babel: Words and the Way We See Things* (Viking, New York: 2001).

John McWhorter, *The Power of Babel: A Natural History of Language* (Perennial, New York: 2001).

Most intriguing, even enthralling in some ways, are the following two books on language by Guy Deutscher which I was unable to put down: *The Unfolding of Language: The Evolution of Mankind's Greatest Invention* (William Heinemann, Random House, London: 2005) and *Through the Language Glass: Why the World Looks Different in Other Languages* (William Heinemann, Random House, London: 2010).

Further information on anatomy, embryology, medicine and surgery is available in countless manuals and it is not my intention to encourage the consultation of any particular one. Other subjects such as the genetics of deafness are too much on the move for books and anyone specially interested should look to the internet and scientific journals.

Likewise, speech pathology and speech therapy is an important academic profession with its own literature and I would hardly presume to give recommendations there. What I have written is intended to be enough to represent my purpose.

What I have written on disease and on the surgery of deafness is based entirely on my own experience and only I am responsible for what I have said.

Index

Printed in the United States
By Bookmasters